HOW TO THRIVE, NOT JUST SURVIVE

A Guide to Developing Independent Life Skills for Blind and Visually Impaired Children and Youths

Rose-Marie Swallow, Ed.D.,
and Kathleen Mary Huebner, Ph.D.,
Editors

Preface by Susan Jay Spungin, Ed.D.

PRESS
New York

HOW TO THRIVE, NOT JUST SURVIVE
A Guide to Developing Independent Life Skills
for Blind and Visually Impaired Children and Youths

Copyright © 1987 by
American Foundation for the Blind
11 Penn Plaza
New York, NY 10001

The American Foundation for the Blind—the organization to which Helen Keller devoted over 40 years of her life—is a national nonprofit whose mission is to eliminate the inequities faced by the ten million Americans who are blind or visually impaired. Headquartered in New York City, AFB maintains offices in Atlanta, Chicago, Dallas, and San Francisco, and a governmental relations office in Washington, DC. For more information, visit: www.afb.org.

PHOTO CREDITS

AFB, pp. 7, 9, 10; Jane Evelyn Atwood, Perkins School for the Blind, p. 5; J. A. Bensel, Maryland School for the Blind, pp. 2, 11, 17, 25, 28, 37, 42, 50, 52; Ann Grady, Perkins School for the Blind, p. 57; Bradford F. Herzog, pp. 15, 62; Ray "Scotty" Morris, cover, p. 20; Brian Mortimer, Baltimore Sunpapers, p. 68; New Mexico School for the Visually Handicapped, cover, pp. 31, 63, 65, 71, 73, 76; Perkins School for the Blind, p. 38; Wisconsin School for the Visually Handicapped, cover, pp. 19, 22, 23, 34, 36, 41, 60, 70

Library of Congress Cataloging-in-Publication Data
How to thrive, not just survive.
Bibliography: p.
1. Children, Blind—United States—Life skills guides.
2. Visually handicapped children—United States—Life skills guides.
I. Swallow, Rose-Marie. II. Huebner, Kathleen Mary.
HV1795.H68   1987   362.4'1'088056 87-12634
ISBN 0-89128-148-7

Printed in the United States of America

CONTENTS

FOREWORD

How to Thrive, Not Just Survive is the result of several years' work by more than 30 professionals brought together by the American Foundation for the Blind. These professionals sought to present, in one comprehensive book, guidelines and strategies to help blind and visually impaired youngsters to develop, acquire, and apply skills they need for independence in daily living, orientation and mobility, and leisure-time and recreational activities. The aim was to reach the wide audience of parents, teachers, and all others involved in the education of these children.

That these professionals succeeded so admirably in completing a formidable task is a testament to their perseverance and dedication to our common goal, a meaningful and dignified life for all blind and visually impaired people.

William F. Gallagher, M.S.W.
Executive Director
American Foundation for the Blind

PREFACE

Over the years, people in the field of education of visually handicapped children and youths have come to appreciate that the education of these children consists of more than just the traditional academic curriculum of reading, writing, and arithmetic. There has been growing concern toward addressing the unique needs of this population, specifically the communication areas in light of advancing technology. Where we as a field continue to fall short, however, is in the area of social and emotional development as it relates to daily living skills, orientation and mobility, and recreation. One of the barriers to progress has been the lack of teaching materials and designated persons whose responsibility it is to address these areas as well as where the actual learning should take place.

How to Thrive is thus designed as a resource in self-help skills, orientation and mobility, and recreation for all those professionals, parents, and significant others who have the potential to have a positive impact on how their visually handicapped learners acquire these basic skills.

The American Foundation for the Blind realized the need for such a book and brought together two groups of professionals to address these issues from the perspective of a visually handicapped child in a mainstreamed setting as well as a visually handicapped child in a residential school. It soon became clear that many of the curriculum needs and methods were the same, and therefore the two manuscripts were combined into one. It gives me great pleasure to see this important publication now available and I wish to take this opportunity to thank not only Dr. Rose-Marie Swallow and Dr. Kathleen Mary Huebner, who served as the final editors on the project, but also all those other hardworking individuals listed below.

Henry A. Aldridge; Polly Amrein; Fred Baker; Bob Brasher; Ralph Brewer; Pat Carpenter; Marcia J. Carter, Re.D.; Anne L. Corn, Ed.D.; Charlyn Sirmans Culver; Dennis Duda; Sara Fogg; John Gunia; Herbert J. Huebner; Ruth Holmes; M. Diane Klein, Ph.D.; Paul T. Lewis; Leslie Machov; Shelly Maron, Ph.D.; Dennis G. McGough, ACSW; Susan Miller; Purvis Ponder; Michael Scione; Rona Shaw, Ed.D.; Janet Simon, Ph.D.; Audrey Smith; Janet Stenson; Betsy Hatlen Wada; Marion V. Wurster, ACSW.

Susan Jay Spungin, Ed.D.,
Associate Executive Director for Program Services
American Foundation for the Blind

PURPOSE

This book provides information about the needs of blind and visually impaired youngsters. It presents guidelines and strategies for helping these children to develop as well as acquire and apply skills that are necessary for independence in socialization, orientation and mobility, and leisure-time and recreational activities. It is designed for all who are involved in the education of blind and visually impaired children: parents and other family members; teachers' aides; houseparents; child care workers; regular classroom teachers; support staff members, such as community home workers, physical and occupational therapists; rehabilitation teachers and counselors; and special education teachers of various disciplines.

The information that is included is applicable to blind and visually impaired infants, children, and adolescents, as well as to children who have mildly concomitant handicapping conditions accompanying this sensory loss. It does not directly address the needs of children who are severely/profoundly mentally and physically handicapped or the unique skills and techniques needed to teach them. However, if such children have a vision loss, the principles of learning presented here can be applied to them. A list of resources is provided for those readers who seek more in-depth information on any of the three independent life skill areas addressed in this book.

Rose-Marie Swallow
Kathleen Mary Huebner

Part I
DAILY LIVING SKILLS

INTRODUCTION

Parents of blind or visually impaired children frequently ask:

How will I help my child learn self-help skills?

Will my child be able to function independently?

Am I doing the right things?

What can I do to help my child become as independent as possible?

Will my child be accepted as an equal in society or treated differently as a disabled person?

These questions and others express the concerns and anxieties of parents, house-parents, and teachers of visually impaired children. It is important to remember that there is no one correct way to rear blind or visually impaired children. Each child has different needs. Therefore, encouraging the development of self-help and personal management skills must take into consideration the needs, requirements, and culture of the individual child. This manual contains practical suggestions and functional techniques which have been gathered from field experiences with parents and children, for helping blind and visually impaired children learn critically needed skills.

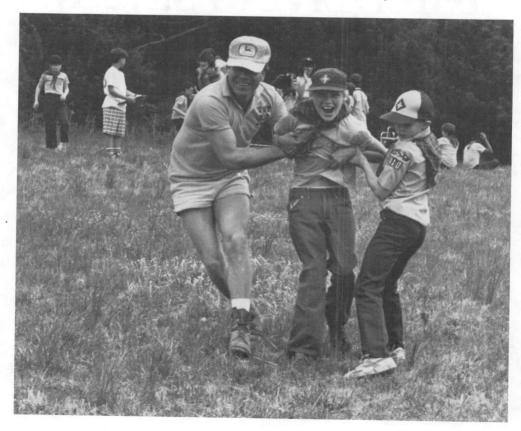

Some definitions

Sighted children learn social skills by watching and listening to others in their environment. The socialization of blind and visually impaired children can be limited because the loss of vision affects their ability to benefit from observing many types of interactions and the subtle nuances of social behavior.

Meaningful social experiences are those in which children actively participate and interact with others. Adults are the primary models for learning to do so, and the quality of the interaction depends on their understanding of and the ability to teach these children. Thus, it is not enough simply to interact. Adult models must recognize the children's needs, anticipate how to meet those needs, routinely and consistently instruct the children, and provide sufficient opportunities for learning.

Because blind and visually impaired children cannot observe others performing an activity, and because some skills are more difficult to observe or learn with limited vision, it takes longer for them than for sighted children to acquire personal management skills. Hence, direct instruction, often involving physical manipulation, must begin as soon as an individual child is ready. **Age-appropriate** is a term used throughout this manual. It means that children should be physically, mentally, and emotionally ready to learn and use a skill. It also means that if a particular skill needs to be developed, activities selected to teach the skill should be similar to those generally performed by children of a similar chronological age.

Therefore, a child's development is an indicator of when a particular skill should be introduced. It must be kept in mind that too much pressure often produces resistance or feelings of inadequacy that may inhibit the child's development. Thus, progress should be carefully noted because it may provide a basis for a realistic evaluation of the child's rate of learning, of when to reward, or when changes, modifications, support, and encouragement are needed.

Independence is the ability to meet one's needs to cope with one's environment, and to control one's life. Independence affords freedom and choice. Learning the skills that foster independence begins at birth and continues throughout life. For blind and visually impaired children to be independent, they must be able to learn and to make appropriate decisions. Only with the development of an effective personal management system will they have the ability to choose how, when, and where to use certain skills. Since the acquisition of most skills is developmental and hence dependent on maturation and past learning experiences, the time to initiate social learning is when a skill is age-appropriate for a child and applicable to everyday situations.

Most skills are more readily learned if a child has had **"hands-on"** experiences; that is, the child's hands are guided through the the tasks of feeding, dressing, and bathing. The child experiences the actions while the adult physically guides and verbalizes the acts. The adult places the child's hands and arms over or under his or hers and guides the child through the entire act. Often it is helpful if the adult works from behind the child rather than facing the child so that the child can feel the arms as well as the hands, the legs as well as the feet, and so forth.

It is also important to encourage **self-initiated** and **discovery learning**. If visual verification is limited or impossible, the child may not be able to judge his or her success, which makes verbal feedback essential. Learning experiences should be pleasant, fun, and rewarding. The blind child needs verbal verification and demonstrations of affection throughout the learning process, whether the experiences involve direct teaching or are initiated by the child. Eventually, the child should learn to evaluate the quality of his or her performance through nonvisual sensory cues.

How skills are acquired and taught

Initially, a young child cannot be expected to appreciate the value of such self-help skills as clean clothes or groomed hair. Such personal values normally emerge after the technique is learned, the physical change that results from the activity is recognized, and the social value of the skill is appreciated. Later, the child incorporates such skills into a personal value system. The sequence for the development of daily living skills most often follows 1) learning a specific skill, 2) the incorporation of the skill into a daily routine, and 3) application of the skill as needed.

When teaching a skill, adults should be thoroughly familiar with it and should break the task into small, sequential steps. The task must be adapted to the child's level of ability but, over time, all the critical components must be taught. Improvement will be noted as the child grows physically and mentally through this experience.

Although the adult may have a preferred method for accomplishing a particular task, the child should be encouraged to discover the most efficient and reasonable way to perform it because the only criteria for tasks are that they should be performed in a safe, efficient, independent, and traditional manner. The adult must be sensitive to the child's desire for experimentation and need for adaptation, as well as to any social and cultural differences. Variations in specific sequences and techniques should be permitted as long as the basic criteria for performing tasks are met. Much of the security that visually impaired adults feel and that permits them to venture into new learning experiences has its beginning in childhood—through the early learning of self-management skills and the acceptance of responsibility.

Young blind and visually impaired children do not learn basic personal and travel management skills incidentally. Therefore, a structured program that provides systematic and consistent instruction is necessary. During such instruction, it is particularly important that the time and place be appropriate to the specific task being taught. For example, dressing skills are best taught in the morning and in the bedroom or bathroom, and toilet training should take place in the bathroom even though it may be more convenient to place the potty in another room. Children need to learn not only when and where it is appropriate to perform certain tasks but also the purpose and function of various rooms and how to get to and from them. Most often, the natural environment is the best place to teach a specific skill.

Another crucial requirement for teaching tasks to young visually impaired and blind children is that sufficient time must be spent on the tasks. It is frequently easier for a harried adult to say, "I'll do it for you because we're in a hurry." However, if the child is not given the time to learn a task, the child will soon be past the age when he or she should have become independent in that skill. The lack of independence in daily living skills can be an embarrassment to the child and can subject the child to ridicule by other children.

Because the ability to perform self-help skills is necessary for the development of self-confidence and self-esteem, it is essential that the visually impaired child be motivated and encouraged to develop a personal management system and taught how to do so.

Finally, visually impaired children will encounter many frustrating situations, which should be dealt with as they occur so they learn how to deal appropriately with frustration. Calm, gentle, and constructive help should be provided. After a frustrating episode, the adult should discuss with the child alternative ways to solve specific problems.

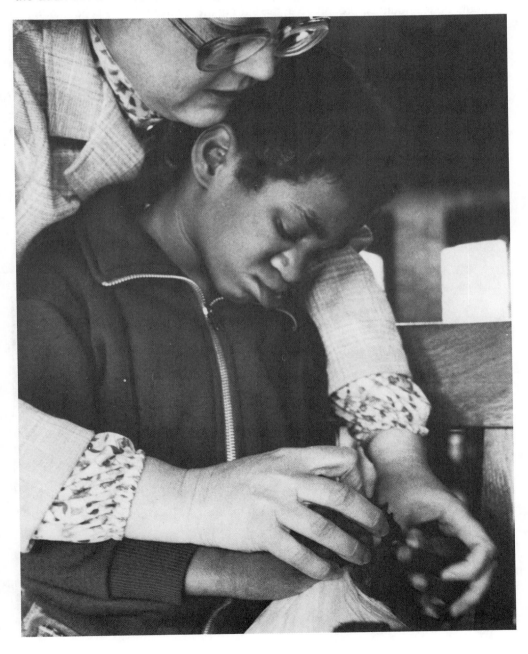

EATING

Many young blind and visually impaired children have to be shown finger feeding as well as the basic motions of chewing if they cannot observe an adult. As feeding progresses past the bottle stage, eating skills are taught at mealtime. Unfamiliar and more difficult foods should be presented at the start of the meal when the child is hungrier and more highly motivated.

If possible, eating skills should be taught at the table when the rest of the family is eating. It is important for the child to learn the social aspects of mealtime in addition to the physical skills involved in eating. However, in the beginning, it may be easier for cleaning up and ultimately better for learning if the child is taught how to eat at a different time. The child needs time to explore foods—to feel their texture and recognize their various states (raw, cooked, mashed). This learning experience can be messy, but it is important.

Finger feeding can be taught by gently guiding the child's hand to the food and simultaneously explaining what it is and how it should be eaten. Bite-size pieces of food, such as cheese and meat, should be placed on the tray of the high chair, and

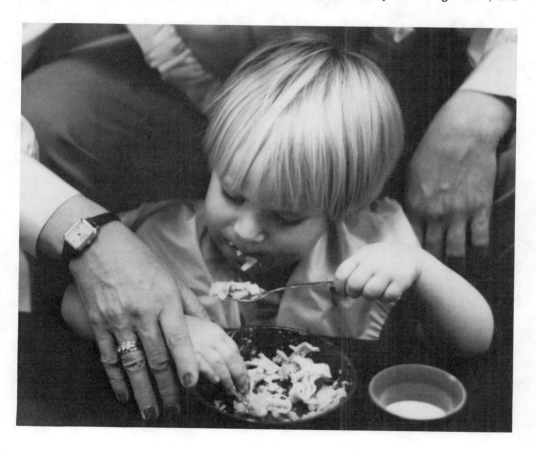

the child should be directed to explore the surface to locate them. Guide the throughout the process, even helping to bring the food to the child's mouth. If use food that the child is particularly fond of, he will be motivated to learn because the food will be pleasurable.

After the child becomes proficient at finger feeding, she should be taught how to use a spoon independently. While sitting or standing behind the child, reach around and place your hand and arm either over or under the child's with the spoon grasped by both of you. This technique helps the child feel the complete motion of holding and lifting the spoon, reaching and scooping food, and placing it so it reaches the mouth. The same technique is used for drinking from a cup or a glass. Place your hands over or under the child's hands, grasp the cup, and show the child how to lift the cup, drink from it, and place it on the tray.

Initially, bowls should be used for self-feeding; the child should then progress to partitioned dishes and finally to standard dishes. By the time the child enters elementary school, he should be using spoons and forks, standard dishes, and possibly knives.

Encourage the child to use a piece of bread or cracker as a "pusher" to secure the food on the fork. A careful scooping motion toward the pusher held away from the edge of the plate enables the child to keep food from sliding off the plate. In addition, the knife should be introduced as early as possible. The preferred method of cutting and eating with a knife and fork is the continental method because it is less cumbersome, involves fewer steps, and eliminates having to relocate the cut piece of food before eating it. With the continental method, the fork is kept in the same hand throughout the process of cutting and eating. The knife is held in the dominant hand and is used both to cut and to secure food on the fork. This method should be taught the same way as is done for other techniques—by placing your hand over or under the child's hands.

General stages of feeding

Accepting the bottle, sucking, and swallowing
Attempting to hold the bottle
Holding the bottle independently
Fingering the food but not lifting it to the mouth
Fingering the food and sucking or tonguing it without chewing
Chewing textured food
Finger feeding and chewing food
Manipulating a spoon and a cup or a glass

Spoon feeding and drinking with assistance
Spoon feeding and drinking independently using one hand
Washing hands before and after meals with help
Washing hands independently before and after meals
Using a fork
Using a knife
Pouring liquids into a glass

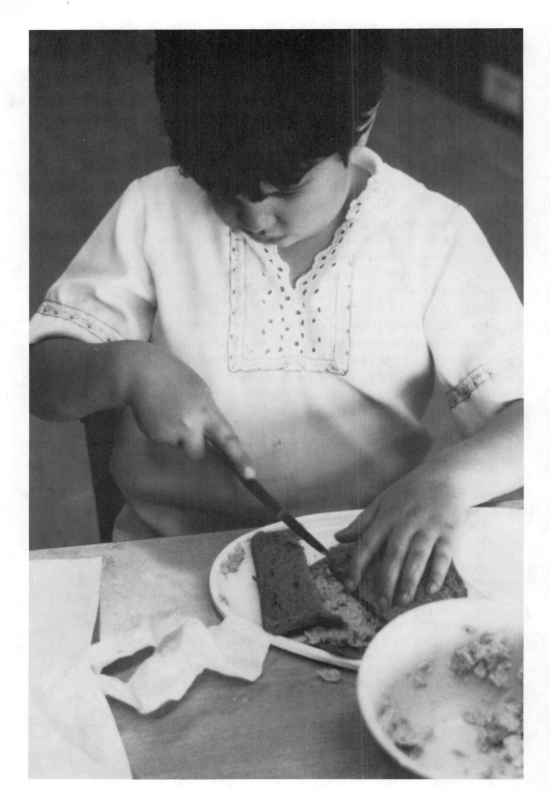

TOILETING

Two major factors should be kept in mind when teaching a child to use the toilet. First, all the adults involved in the process should use consistent language, techniques, and procedures. Second, a routine schedule should be followed, developed from the child's personal needs and daily routines. Generally, if meals are consumed at certain times, the child will need to eliminate at approximately the same time each day. This routine may be more difficult to achieve with some children, and consultation with the child's physician may be necessary.

Before toilet training begins, record the times when the child eliminates and how long the child stays dry and try to determine the child's natural pattern of behavior. Consistently use preselected words for "dryness" or "wetness," (the same holds true for bowel movements). The objective is for the child to know "wetness," which aids in anticipating that he is about to urinate. Unless the child becomes aware of internal signals, he is not learning.

The toileting sequence

Sits on the potty for a short time

Sits on the potty for a longer period

Indicates that something has happened or performs on the potty when placed there

Remains dry until placed on the potty or asked to go to the toilet

Goes to the toilet alone

Indicates in some manner that he or she needs to go to the toilet

Remains dry all night

Takes care of the hygienic aspects of toileting

Washes and dries hands after toileting

If male, knows how to stand to urinate

Throughout the toilet training program, the blind child's hands are involved in the process; the child feels the potty chair; places hands on the adult's hands while pulling down pants; uses the adult's hands as a guide while wiping; and, finally, with help, washes and dries hands. Small boys often have difficulty learning how to stand to urinate. Using a tin can initially leads to later understanding of how to target the toilet bowl. If the child wants to touch the bowel movement, do not be upset. Allow the child to do so to satisfy the child's curiosity but do not permit it to become part of the toileting routine.

DRESSING AND UNDRESSING

Independent dressing and undressing skills can considerably shorten the time that parents must spend helping their children. Again, it is important to resist the temptation to dress and undress a child because it is faster to do so rather than to teach the child how to perform these tasks.

If parents begin when the child is very young, by talking about what they are doing (for example, "Give me your hand; now put your arm in the sleeve and push it all the way through"), the child will begin to learn the concepts of clothing and body parts, as well as understand the actions and movements that are involved in dressing. When the child indicates an interest in being independent, begin by teaching the child how to undress, since it is easier to remove clothing than to put it on. The child is likely to become less frustrated if she learns to undress before dressing, unbutton before buttoning, and unzip before zipping.

Develop routines for taking off shoes or socks or a sweater or a coat at appropriate times. Encourage the child to help pull down and pull up pants during toilet training. Begin by using loose-fitting clothes that are the easiest to put on, such as pants with elastic waistbands rather than zippers.

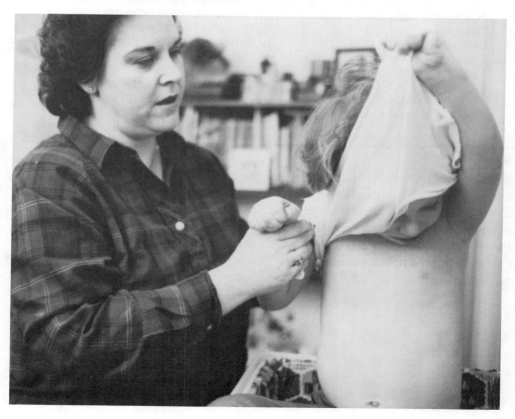

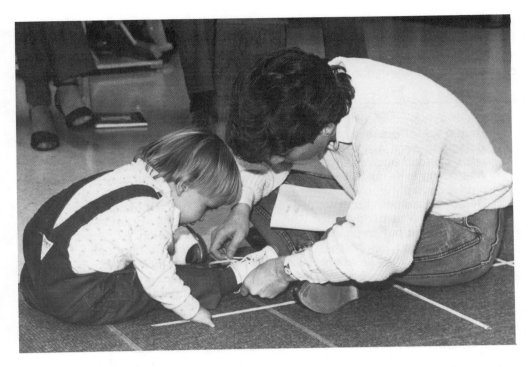

The child also needs to learn how to organize clothing. Set an example by keeping clothes organized in wardrobes, drawers, and closets. Have the child identify which garments are needed, locate where they are stored, and place them on the bed or another flat surface. Lay out garments, tee shirts, pants, and so forth in the order in which they will be put on. Teach the child how to locate the right garments, check that they are right side out, put them on, and smooth them, so they are not twisted on the body. Eventually, you may discuss color coordination and the general principles of style.

Children can become familiar with the concepts of laterality (right and left) before or while they learn to put on their shoes and can be taught to insert the correct foot into the correct shoe and to pull up the tongue, if necessary. Different tactile markings on the soles of shoes help to identify right and left. Shoes with Velcro fasteners or slip-on shoes, such as loafers, are much easier. However, if the child is physically able, shoe-tying skills should be taught as well.

Shoe-tying skills require fine motor development and thus generally are learned after the child enters elementary school. Shoe models or adult shoes are helpful while teaching lacing and knot tying. They should be placed in front of the child with the heel closest to him so the shoe is in the position it would be if it were on the child. Work on the lace first. Make one shoelace by tying together two laces in contrasting colors and/or laces with two textures and center the laces between the bottom eyelets. In teaching the child how to tie laces, place the shoe on a table or wrap the laces around the child's thigh with the ends on top, so they can be tied on top of the thigh.

Buttoning and zipping also help to develop motor control. Begin by using large buttons on loose-fitting garments and zippers on pants or skirts that do not need to be threaded. By the time the child enters elementary school, she should be able to put on, fasten, and remove pants, shirts, coats, and sweaters with little help. During the preschool years, emphasize dressing skills using self-help teaching materials and equipment. Unless you begin to teach these techniques early, you will find that the child may be old enough for school but cannot put on her clothing.

Sequence of dressing and undressing skills

Extending arms when being dressed and undressed

Attempting to remove clothes independently

Removing clothes that have pull-on elastic waistbands

Attempting to put on simple, loose clothing with help

Putting on clothes independently

Attempting to remove a sweater or unbutton a coat

Helping to unbutton a coat

Unbuttoning a coat

Attempting to unzip clothing

Unzipping clothing

Zipping zippers that do not require threading

Attempting to start unthreaded zippers with help

Attempting to start unthreaded zippers independently

Starting unthreaded zippers and zipping independently

Putting on clothes if they are handed to him

Identifying articles of clothing and knowing the order in which clothes are put on

Distinguishing the front and back and the inside and outside of garments and turning the garments to the correct side

Differentiating the left from the right side of clothes and shoes

Dressing independently

Selecting a complete outfit from drawers and a closet

Selecting clothing that is appropriate to the weather or season

Folding, hanging, and storing clothes

MOTOR DEVELOPMENT

Activities that stress the use and coordination of the large and small muscles are necessary if the child is to perform such **gross motor activities** as sitting, walking, and playing and such **fine motor activities** as grasping, releasing objects, dressing, cutting, and writing.

The development of large body movements may be encouraged by getting on the floor with the child and helping him roll and crawl, and by directing and making the initial motions for the child (for instance, left hand and right knee forward, then right hand and left knee forward). Plan games that involve a mixture of locomotion skills, walking, running, hopping, skipping, jumping, sliding, and so forth. Use gymnastic equipment, such as balls and scooter boards, and set up obstacle courses that encourage the use of large and small body movements. In addition, plan activities that require the child to pick up and squeeze objects of different sizes and textures, including balls, bean bags, and stuffed toys. Encourage the child to learn how to operate mechanical toys.

First, go through the motions with the child and then ask the child to perform these activities independently. Such activities as screwing tops on containers, placing beads in jars, and making shapes with Lego blocks and clay develop fine motor control. Select activities that are meaningful and those in which the child can feel he is accomplishing something.

Balance

Natural movement requires the constant changing of body positions and the ability to maintain equilibrium and coordinate all motions. To develop good balance, the child should first stand on two feet and then one foot while extending the arms to the side. At first, the child should stand on the floor or another stable surface. Then she can try to stand on an unstable surface, such as a trampoline or inner tube. Initially, the child can use the arms to maintain balance if there is a solid object such as parallel bars on either side or a wall to one side. As the child becomes more secure in balancing, gently push the child off balance so she can learn to fall or regain balance independently.

Community centers and schools often have skilled staff members, such as adaptive physical education teachers and physical therapists, who can provide guidance and design specific activities that utilize specialized equipment to develop balancing skills. Keep in mind that all adults who work with the child must routinely and consistently communicate with each other if the child is to learn as much as he is able.

Posture

The early emphasis on good posture will help the child move more efficiently and prevent poor postural habits that will be difficult to correct later. Therefore, the blind and visually impaired infant should be guided to assume different postures (such as sitting, rolling over, and standing). You can help the infant become familiar with many body positions while playing with toys that produce sound: instead of handing the toys to her, place them in different locations to encourage shifts in body movements and posture. Play hide-and-seek with noise-making toys.

Encourage the child to hold the head erect and provide verbal feedback and physical assistance to correct the position of head, trunk, and extremities. Tell the child when she is demonstrating poor as well as good posture and help the child monitor her own movements. Some children may position their heads high or to the side in an attempt to use their remaining vision more efficiently. Familiarize yourself with the child's best visual field of view before requiring any change in the position of the head. Consult an occupational or physical therapist when physical limitations or complications are present. If a child requires adaptive equipment, it is important that this be provided and used correctly.

Gait and stride

Many blind and visually impaired children will need guidance and feedback about the appropriateness and consistency of their gait and stride. To correct these problems, walk with the child or place the child's feet on your feet, then adjust the length of your stride to the child's size and stride.

Some blind or visually impaired children will pull back or lunge forward while walking with a sighted guide. Discuss the effects of these actions and help the child become aware of this way of walking. Be sure to give the child positive reinforcement when he walks correctly. Since the correct use of a sighted guide is such an important part of socialization, it is important that the child learn how to walk correctly so as not to put undue tension on the guide's body.

Integration of body movements

The visually impaired child needs to use her remaining senses (including vision) and to maintain a general awareness of the body while engaged in basic movements such as walking before learning more advanced movements and travel skills. In the beginning, provide a safe, uncluttered environment so the child will feel secure about moving. If doors are left open and unexpected objects lying around, the child will not feel safe enough to move into the environment or explore her surroundings.

When the child is motivated to move and feels secure about moving, introduce a variety of activities and experiences such as walking independently on slopes and up and down stairs. Encourage the child to alternate feet on stairs while holding the handrail. While walking, guide the child's coordination of her foot movements and arm swings to maintain good balance and present a pleasing appearance.

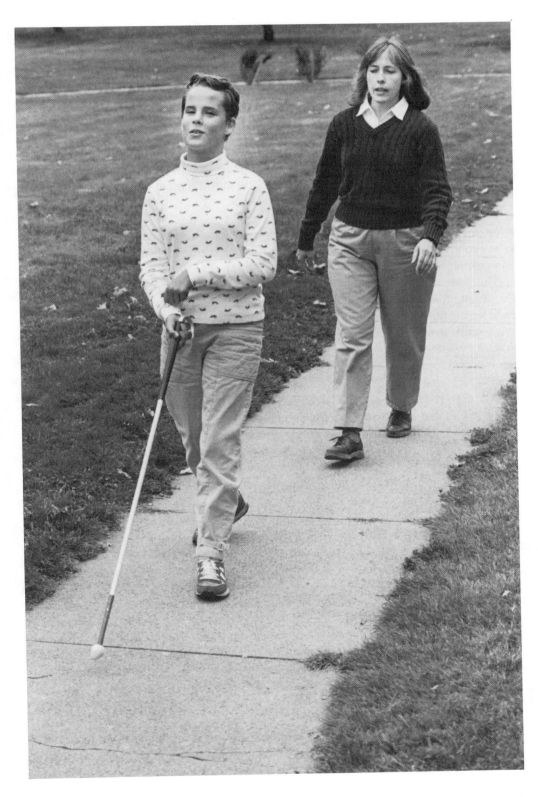

LEARNING TO BE INDEPENDENT

Children usually enjoy helping Mommy and Daddy. Blind and visually impaired children also enjoy doing so but they may have little awareness of what "helping" is about and will need to be encouraged and instructed in these skills. Parents need to take advantage of the children's eagerness to participate and use the opportunity to teach them how to be independent. Effective learning takes place when children are having fun. The following are a few skills that may be introduced in this manner.

Finding Mom and Dad

When the mother or father is not within hearing distance, the child should be encouraged to do a room-to-room search, politely calling out for Mom or Dad. In the beginning, when one parent is with the child, he should ask, "Where's Mommy?" and then say, "Let's find her." He should then take the child through an appropriate room-to-room search. Eventually, the child will seek and locate the parent independently. In this process, the child learns not only the pattern of how to search but how he needs to move in addition to meeting his needs and feeling a sense of accomplishment. It is important for parents to recognize and take advantage of such natural learning situations. Doing so eliminates aggravation and frustration and the need to create contrived situations.

How to play with, pick up, and put away toys

When presented with a new toy, the child first needs to be given a chance to explore and experiment with it using her hands and mouth. Many youngsters like to mouth toys and objects. This is okay in order to gain information about the toy, but should not be a part of the playing routine. The parent should explain to the child how the toy works, what it does, what it is called, and how to use it. Together they can learn about and have fun with the toy.

Each toy should have its own storage space. At an early age, visually impaired and blind children can start helping by putting a favorite toy in a special place. Helping hands and encouraging voices guide them across the room to the shelf where the toy goes. As they mature and gain confidence, they can be given responsibility for more toys and objects.

Visually impaired or blind children should be taught to locate lost or dropped objects. As soon as they drop an object, toddlers must learn to listen for and localize the sound of the object as it hits the surface and trace the sound of the object as it rolls or bounces. Then they should kneel and begin a slow systematic search of the area. If they get discouraged, the adult should gently encourage them and give them directions on how to locate the object. Locating objects can be fun if the adult makes a game of it.

Putting away clothes

In teaching children to put away clothes in their proper place, one strategy is to fold clothes together into "outfits" and place them in a plastic dishpan when they are removed from the dryer or clothesline. The children can then carry the pan to their room, remove

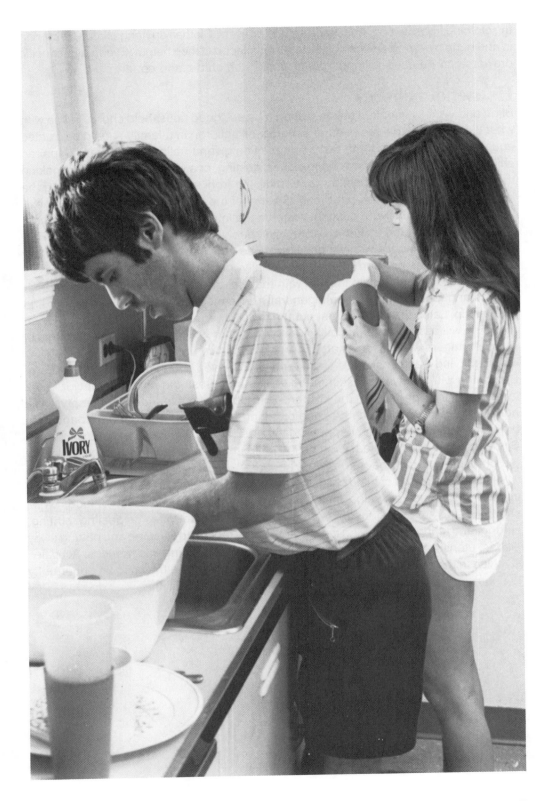

the clothing from the pan, and place it in the drawers. Clothes on hangers can be carried in and hung by young children on a closet rod placed at their height. Eventually, specific drawers can be used for underpants, socks, tee shirts, and so forth.

Household chores

Blind and visually impaired children should be assigned household chores in line with what is normally expected of other siblings. All children in a family should be treated equally within reason. Some tasks that may be given to blind and visually impaired children include washing and drying dishes, dusting, or sweeping, vacuuming, making the bed, emptying wastebaskets, sweeping the front walk, raking leaves, doing the laundry, and helping to prepare food. Several of these tasks will be discussed next. While you are vacuuming, dusting, sweeping, allow the child to work alongside you, "helping" to push the vacuum, carpet sweeper, or broom, and to hold the dust rag. Since the child cannot visually observe these activities, by helping he learns that household chores are part of everyone's daily routine.

The child must become familiar with these cleaning utensils to learn about their actions and functions. Real items generally have meaning before toy sweepers and brooms do. Later, the child will get out the toy cleaners "to help" clean house. Eventually, he will assume responsibility for specific chores. Remember, the bedrooms of most teenagers are "disaster areas," but do not give up.

Emptying wastebaskets is a simple task that even young children can perform. Beginning with the wastebasket in the child's room, ask the child to empty it into a larger container, perhaps in the kitchen. This job can be expanded into emptying all household baskets into a central one or taking the baskets out to the garbage can, bin or incerator chute. What happens to the trash should be explained and observed. Since this task is usually easy for a blind child, make sure that it is not the only duty the child performs in the home.

Visually impaired or blind children should be encouraged to participate with adults in meal preparation activities, including menu planning; the selection of foods while shopping; the storage of foods; such food preparation activities as peeling, cutting, stirring, and frying; and serving meals. Setting the table and washing and putting away dishes, utensils, and pots and pans can be excellent learning experiences. Activities involved in the preparation of meals can be fun and can give the child an opportunity to share in the family's activities and to assume responsibilities.

PERSONAL HYGIENE AND GROOMING

To lead independent lives, blind and visually impaired children and youths must incorporate the skills necessary to maintain an acceptable level of personal hygiene and grooming. All children need to be taught specific grooming skills, such as the proper use of a washcloth and how to soap, rinse, and dry their bodies. Personal cleanliness, proper hygienic care of body parts and prosthetic devices, and the ability to take medicine or to apply first-aid treatment are important to the maintenance of health, fitness, and vitality. Some children need to be reminded or encouraged to improve specific grooming and hygiene skills. There are a number of specific skills that children should learn through direct instruction and intervention by adults.

Hand and face care

Orienting self to sink, soap and towel areas

Regulating water temperature

Wetting, soaping, lathering, and washing hands

Wetting and soaping washcloth

Using washcloth to soap face and neck

Using washcloth to soap face and neck

Thoroughly rinsing hands and face

Wringing dry and hanging washcloth

Drying hands and face

Hanging up towel

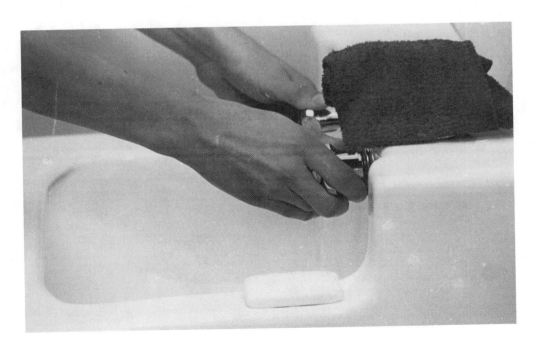

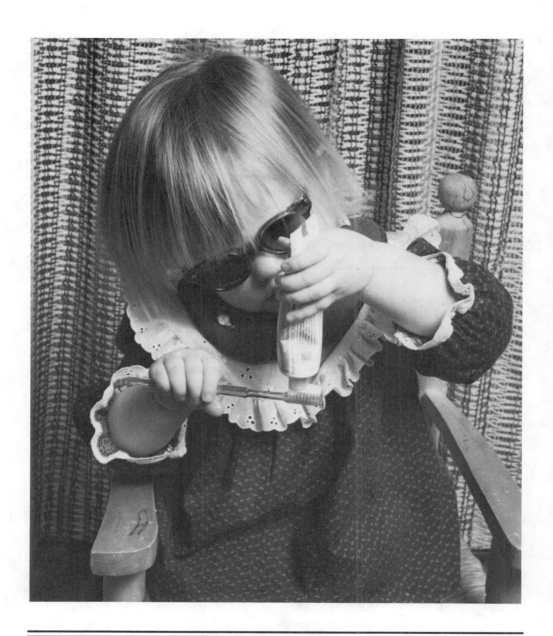

Hair care

Combing, parting, and brushing the hair

Washing the hair

Arranging the hair in an attractive style using hair-styling devices and appliances

Making appropriate grooming decisions about cutting and styling the hair

Going to the barber shop or beauty salon

Dental care
Brushing the teeth, using the
  correct movement
Applying the correct amount of
  toothpaste to the toothbrush
Putting away the toothbrush and
  toothpaste

Rinsing the mouth well
  with mouthwash
Using dental floss
Applying proper eating habits to
  maintain the teeth
Having regular dental checkups

Nail care
Cleaning and brushing the nails
Cutting and shaping the nails
Using an emery board
  and nail file

Caring for the cuticles and
  preventing hangnails
Maintaining hand
  and foot hygiene

Showering independently
Safely regulating the water
  temperature
Wetting and soaping the
  washcloth
Soaping the entire body,
  including the eyes, ears, and
  genital areas

Thoroughly rinsing the body
Drying the body
Hanging up the washcloth
Replacing soiled towels
Leaving the bathroom in a
  sanitary and orderly condition

Skin care
Putting on clean clothing after
  bathing
Removing unwanted hair

Using a deodorant, creams or
  lotions, ointments or salves

Of course, young children may not need all the skills listed. However, at the appropriate age, children require specific directions so they may learn selected grooming skills. Therefore, professionals and parents must take care that appropriate learning opportunities have been presented. (See the available resources for independent living skills that are listed at the end of this guide.)

CHOICE AND CARE OF CLOTHING

Successful participation in society requires an awareness of current clothing styles. Although it is often suggested that there is a wide range of acceptable clothing, in practice this is not true. Since this society contains many subgroups, each of which often has its own style, to be a member of a subgroup one must conform to a recognizable standard of dress. Thus, blind and visually impaired children need to be aware of and be able to conform to various standards or codes of dress so they will have the freedom to choose the group to which they wish to belong, and parents should understand the importance of personal appearance for creating social interaction.

As a rule, schools do not have a strict dress code. However, clothing needs to fit properly and should be clean and free of rips and stains. Visually impaired and blind children should not be sent to school in unattractive clothing or clothing that is not typical of the attire worn by their peers.

Furthermore, visually impaired children should participate in choosing their clothes. Many factors bear on the selection of clothing. Whether the clothing is new or used, its style, how well it fits, and its degree of conformity to the standard of dress required

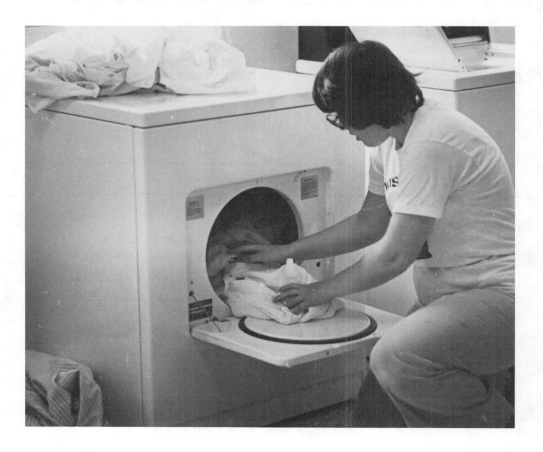

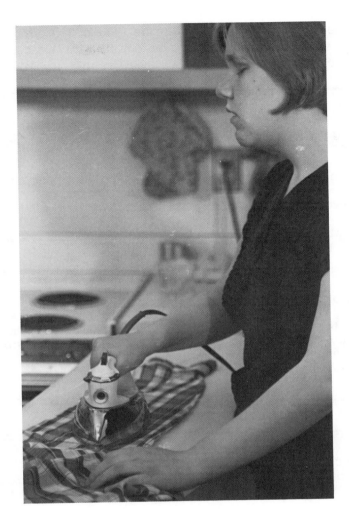

by the social situation should help determine its suitability. Teenagers determine the value of clothes, as well as jewelry, accessories, and makeup, on the basis of what is "in," not on the basis of cost.

Encourage youngsters to seek information from others on their clothing and appearance. "Does this look right?" It might be better to find out that there is a spot on one's clothing before leaving for school or work than to be embarrassed later in the day.

The choice of items depends on the function for which they are intended. The appropriateness of line, color, design, and texture of fabrics depends on the situation in which the clothing will be worn and what complements the child's physical characteristics. Clothing is an important aspect of the overall impression one makes on others. Other people perceive our clothing as a reflection of our personalities, especially how we feel about ourselves; thus, our choice of clothing reflects our self-image and self-esteem.

Extreme styles are inappropriate unless the child has other personal qualities to carry off the effect, such as posture and gait, facial expression, hair style, language patterns, and other affective mannerisms associated with the "look." Styles that are widely accepted by the majority of peers tends to be more useful for developing social contacts. Visually impaired and blind children should develop the facility to recognize styles and to choose and care for their clothes and cosmetics. This ability involves several factors:

Style

Matching proper pieces of clothing in relation to color, patterns and texture

Combining various pieces of clothing to create an attractive outfit

Wearing and combining appropriate accessories to enhance an outfit

Selecting the proper attire for various occasions

Choice of clothes

Selecting styles, colors, and fabrics that are appropriate to one's physical characteristics

Considering the cost, quality, and style of clothes

Choosing outfits that are functionally and socially appropriate for the current fashions and seasons

---

Care of clothes

Folding or hanging one's clothes

Arranging and storing accessories

Caring for and storing clothes

Cleaning and ironing clothes

Cosmetics

Being aware of the style, use, and effects of cosmetics

Selecting and using lotions, shaving products, powders and creams

Storing cosmetics properly and hygienically

Choosing and applying cosmetics, if desired

SOCIALLY APPROPRIATE BEHAVIOR

Although social mores differ from culture to culture and family to family, each society teaches its young certain general rules of behavior to facilitate socialization. Adult workers or teachers of cultures that are different from those of the child need to be familiar with the mores and values of the child's and parents' culture and must adapt their expectations and teaching accordingly. Each child is unique, as is each culture. The way children develop social skills depends on their interactions with others as well as on their personalities. Children may have a variety of behavioral styles in various social situations. Look at whether the child has developed behaviors that are appropriate to situations and that are socially appropriate. It should be noted that there is an extensive repertoire of appropriate and inappropriate behaviors that are judged according to specific situations, rather than in isolation.

Because visual impairment imposes limitations on the amount of experiences and the input received from those experiences, blind and visually impaired children often are not aware of behaviors that they cannot observe. For example, when wearing dresses, young girls learn through observation to sit in certain ways, although they

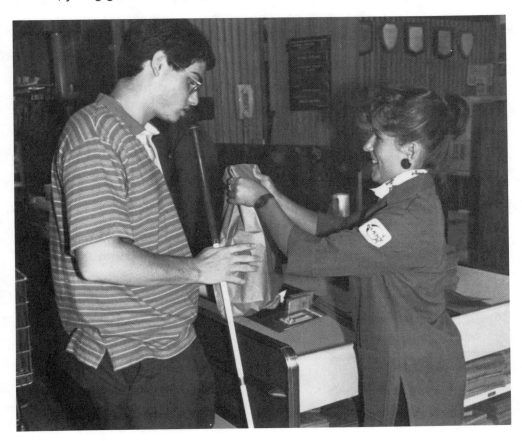

may have to be reminded about the proper positions. Therefore, it is the adult's responsibility to point out socially appropriate ways of handling certain situations when learning through observation is difficult or impossible. Caring adults must inform children when their behaviors are not appropriate and offer them options.

Visually impaired children may sometimes learn actions through observation but, at other times, they seem oblivious to those around them; thus, adults cannot assume that visually impaired youngsters are aware of the behavior of their peers. Furthermore, visual impairment sometimes requires that children use special techniques to function efficiently; for example, a blind child may have to be taught to sprinkle salt or pepper into his or her hand to determine which it is before putting it on the food. Hence, while the child is learning what is socially appropriate, he or she is also learning specific skills that are related to blindness or visual impairment. The child's use of specialized techniques that maximize independence must be respected.

In considering how to help the blind or visually impaired child develop appropriate social skills, adults should consider two points. First, the child should not learn that appearing to be sighted is best, which may lead to a denial of the impairment. However, when the child is old enough to understand the rules governing social interactions, he should be begin to eliminate obtrusive behaviors that impede the development of social relationships. Second, the child should not be led to believe that tactile means should be used only as a last resort. He must feel free to receive information tactually when necessary and appropriate; otherwise, inefficient methods of functioning may develop that could reduce independence.

Stereotypic behavior

Some, but not all, visually impaired and blind children may exhibit stereotypic behaviors that, although not unique to this population, are of concern. Behaviors that are often referred to as "blindisms" may include such repetitive actions as poking and pressing the eyes, rhythmic rocking of the body or head, and finger "flicking." The reasons for these behaviors are not fully understood, but several theories have been explored. For example, it has been suggested that these stereotypic behaviors may represent a way of releasing energy, ignorance of substitute meaningful actions, the need for self-stimulation because of the lack of sensory input, or a way of obtaining information about the environment.

Stereotypic behaviors may be prevented by involving the child in meaningful activities. It is generally accepted that the younger a child is when helped to prevent these behaviors from developing into habits, the easier it is for her to learn new behaviors. Blind children may not be conscious of their mannerisms or that others do not behave in a similar way.

Behavioral change techniques, counseling, and other approaches have been used with various degrees of success to eliminate patterns of stereotypic behaviors. It is recommended that before extreme techniques of behavioral management are considered, some questions should be answered.

It is further recommended that the prevention or elimination of stereotypic behaviors be discussed among all the adults involved in the child's care, particularly the parents and professionals.

Public and private behavior

As children learn socially appropriate behaviors, they may need clarification about when and where to use these behaviors. For example, hair combing, a necessary skill, is inappropriate in a restaurant but acceptable at the beach. Thus, rules of thumb, although helpful to blind and visually impaired children, need to be taught in relation to specific situations.

Each family instructs its children on matters of modesty and privacy, beginning in early childhood, when children first raise questions about sex and the differences between males and females. However, privacy may be a difficult concept for visually impaired children to understand. For example, even though a visually impaired child may be able to see out of the bedroom window to some degree, she may not always be aware that someone can look in the window; therefore, adults need to remind the child to close the drapes or blinds. In addition, it is easy for those who are sighted to find out if another person is nearby before fixing a slip, scratching an itch, and the like, but a visually impaired child must learn to be more cautious in these matters.

Small-group behavior

Blind children do not automatically assume relaxed positions, as sighted children do. They need ample experience and instruction in a variety of casual situations to develop flexible postures.

One important skill is the ability to face the person or persons to whom one is talking. Blind children can learn to do so by localizing sounds and being aware of cues. While developing and practicing conversational skills, they also can be learning appropriate body positions.

Because it is difficult to participate in a group conversation if one is unaware of nonverbal cues, some visually impaired and blind children need to develop conversational techniques. Such factors as when it is appropriate to speak, how to control the level of noise and the direction of the conversation, and when and how to break into a conversation or end it should be discussed in relation to the inflection or direction of the voice and conversational signals. An outgoing, interested personality eases one's entry into new group situations. Although such a personality cannot be taught, group-entry skills can be developed. Practice and participation will further ease the situation.

Shaking hands. Generally, when two people are introduced, they decide if they want to shake hands. However, since a blind or visually impaired child cannot see what the other person is doing, it is better to put the hand out than to leave someone with a hand extended. The child will need to learn the proper way to shake hands—that the arm is extended at about the waist, that the hand is held slightly relaxed, and that the other person's hand is grasped firmly and shaken.

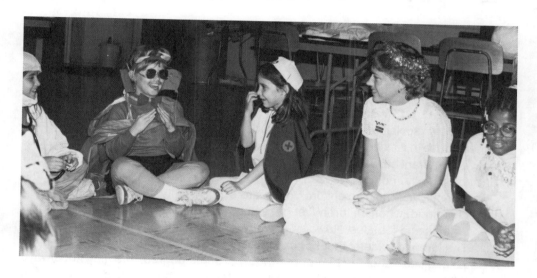

SELF-ESTEEM

Self-images are formed from beliefs about ourselves that are integrated with those that others hold of us. Each blind and visually impaired child needs to feel that he is a worthy and contributing member of the family and the peer group, as well as a unique individual with special talents and abilities. The visual impairment is part of the self and must be incorporated into the total self-image, but it is only one of many attributes, feelings, and emotions. Exaggerated feelings about the limitations imposed by the impairment give it a larger role than it deserves. It is hoped that the child will come to believe that opportunities are opened because of his abilities and not closed because of the impairment.

Relationships with peers

Growing children enter into friendships and associations with people outside their immediate families. Participation in activities with friends and siblings helps them establish new relationships and expand their interactions with others. Adults who realize the need for visually impaired and blind children to be part of the sighted world will arrange for them to have early social experiences with sighted children.

One visually impaired child may live and go to school in a community where she is the only one with a visual impairment. Another may live or go to school with children who have similar disabilities. When visually impaired and blind children have only visually impaired or only sighted friends, they feel forced into accepting the imposed identity group with which they may not feel comfortable.

Visually impaired children may have difficulty identifying with or fitting into social groups of sighted or visually impaired peers. This lack of identity may lead them to develop behavioral patterns in which they attempt to cover up their visual impairment. Some behaviors may be socially acceptable (such as wearing tinted glasses), while others do not serve the student well (not using large-type books in class, for instance). Many of these behaviors reflect strong feelings with which visually impaired children must deal with guidance from emphatic adults. The introduction of these children to successful older visually impaired youngsters and adults is helpful. But, what is of paramount importance is that they learn the techniques of coping with the environment and of controlling social situations.

Adults can help visually impaired children become comfortable in social situations by encouraging them to participate in group activities so they feel they have the right to join groups—the Scouts, church groups, school clubs, etc. They can discuss friendships, the selection of friends, skills to maintain friendships, and why some relationships end. In this regard, puppetry can be a useful tool. Through these discussions, visually impaired children also can begin to place their impairment in perspective and understand that friends are those who can share their experiences—both those that are related to the visual impairments and those that are not. In addition, they can come to understand why peers and adults resort to stereotyping or labeling and find ways to cope with these practices.

Asking for assistance

No one, blind or sighted, is completely independent; we all depend on others. Once skills for independence have been learned, each child must consciously or unconsciously decide how independent he wishes to be. The child who can travel independently may choose to walk with another child for friendship and conversation, but without the ability to move freely such a choice could not be made.

Some children need to be taught how to ask for needed assistance and to refuse unwanted assistance. A visually impaired child who does not appear to have visual problems may be reluctant to ask for assistance. Through role playing, such a child may come to understand the reactions of others and develop appropriate ways to ask for help. "Would you read this price tag to me?" may seem an odd question for someone to ask who does not seem to be visually impaired, but "I can't see the small print on this price tag, could you read it for me?" will explain the situation. Likewise, refusing offered assistance may be done in a positive, nonhostile way so that the helper does not feel snubbed and the child retains a sense of dignity.

Visually impaired children must also learn that they have skills and abilities that they can use to assist others. Participating on a school tutoring team or caring for younger children are two of the many helping activities in which children can engage.

Risk taking

Visually impaired and blind children develop self-esteem in the same way as all children do. Their developing personalities, past experiences, and relationships with others play a part in determining whether they will feel worthy and capable.

Confidence develops through one's recognition of success. Sincere and realistic praise for efforts and accomplishments help one develop positive feelings about oneself. Because visually impaired and blind children experience physical and emotional stress that sighted children do not encounter, they require more encouragement from adults if they are to develop a belief in their abilities, as well as realistic self-expectations which will help to achieve a positive self-concept.

Risk-taking behaviors may be defined as those that are new, are a combination of previously learned behaviors applied to a new situation, and those for which the end result cannot be firmly determined until the deed is accomplished. Although blind and visually impaired children may eagerly anticipate learning a new activity, they may feel anxious about the possibility of unseen hazards in the environment. However, new experiences enable blind and visually impaired children to participate in activities with peers, enhance their coordination, hasten their development of concepts, and lead to new opportunities and feelings of accomplishment. Furthermore, children who have learned to cope with new experiences may be better prepared to perform new tasks in the future because they have gained a sense of security from taking risks and from having been successful or from learning to cope with difficulties.

When blind and visually impaired children begin to engage in activities that involve some risk, many adults will feel anxious, not only because they are afraid that the children will fail or be hurt in the new endeavor but because the consequences of success or failure may create new concerns or changes in routine. For example, once children have learned to cross streets independently, they should be permitted to continue to do so. The anxieties of adults about the children's safety will gradually lessen as the children's success in independent travel increases.

Problem solving

The skills of problem solving go hand in hand with taking risks. When blind and visually impaired children travel independently, they must find solutions to a variety or problems. For example, a teenager who encounters a construction barricade on a familiar walk to school may need to consider a variety of solutions to the problem before he can proceed. A girl whose classmate helper is absent needs to discover another method of obtaining the blackboard notes. Although blind and visually impaired children who come up against expected or unexpected problems may be able to call on others for assistance, they must first know how to communicate their needs. Moreover, when they think they can solve these problems by themselves, they must know how to refuse unnecessary help from overprotective adults.

Adults can be most helpful to visually impaired children by providing them with experiences in which they can learn to solve problems, by discussing alternative solutions, and by guiding the children through thought processes that are involved. As the children become more successful in solving problems, adults can gradually withdraw and decrease their input.

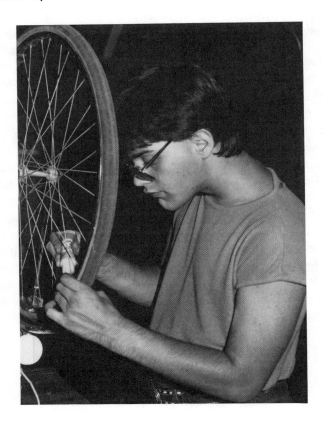

ETIQUETTE

Sighted children learn many techniques of etiquette through direct observation. If they are not sure how to handle a new situation, they can watch others and then duplicate the behavior. However, when visually impaired and blind children enter a new social situation, they may feel awkward unless they have been carefully instructed and have had the opportunity to practice the necessary skills. Even with intensive training, they are bound, sooner or later, to find themselves in a social situation for which they are not prepared. When such a situation arises, a sense of humor, a healthy self-image, and confidence are valuable assets. The following are some specific situations that visually impaired children will encounter and should be taught to handle.

Sneezing, coughing, and yawning. Visually impaired children should be shown how to hold a tissue or handkerchief, apply slight pressure, blow the nose, and wipe it neatly. Covering the mouth while sneezing, coughing, or yawning is also necessary.

Table manners. As other social graces develop, visually impaired and blind children, introduced to various foods and cooking styles, begin to participate in a variety of situations in which eating is a social occasion. The etiquette of eating is acquired through direct instruction, practice, and social awareness, coupled with the desire for social approval. The young child needs careful instruction in eating politely, how to sit, locating items on the plate or table, and which foods to eat with which utensil.

Eating politely involves eating small bits of food, not talking with a full mouth, chewing thoroughly, and inconspicuously removing inedible foods from the mouth. Learning how to identify what is on the plate and where each type of food is located comes from practicing consistently, first at home and then in other settings. The person sitting next to the child quietly describes where each type of food is placed. The common practice is to use the clock method: "Your potatoes are at 11 o'clock and your meat is at 4 o'clock." When teaching the child which utensils to use, adults should describe the types of food that are eaten with each utensil.

Special occasions. Visually impaired and blind children may encounter problems at special occasions such as buffet dinners, salad bars, or picnics. Eating in unfamiliar settings that are basically self-service or where food is served in non-routine ways, such as snacking at parties, teas, and receptions generally requires that participants visually scan the area to locate and identify available foods, serving plates and napkins, if toothpicks are placed in small portions of food, if beverages are self-service and how they are presented, and the like. The blind or visually impaired child should experience all types of social occasions. Adults should describe how things are arranged and the degree of formality or informality of each special occasion and should encourage the child to serve him or herself with verbal (and physical, when necessary) assistance. The child should not be placed in a chair on the sidelines and served. The greater the active participation, the more helpful the experience is to the child's development.

HOME MANAGEMENT

The home provides basic support for living as well as shelter and is the center of daily life. Eating, sleeping, caring for our needs, and socializing all take place at home. Home management is not limited to keeping the house or apartment attractive and orderly, but includes the proper use and care of the materials needed for survival.

It includes such rudimentary tasks as the organization of personal belongings, the care of clothing, bed-making, and dishwashing, and extends to the complicated tasks that are associated with independent adult living.

In most cases, adults should teach children home-management skills that are age-appropriate and that meet the children's immediate needs; they should reinforce these skills daily so they will eventually become self-directed and routine. They must exercise reasonable control so they do not perform the tasks for the children but let the children practice the tasks themselves.

Often, children do not fully appreciate skills until they understand the need for them. This is only possible if the children are permitted to do things for themselves. Therefore, adults should encourage children to realize the need for orderliness and the care of material things, and teach them to perform the necessary skills. Visually impaired children are in no way different from sighted children in their need to acquire home-living skills early in life. However, their dependence on others may be extended beyond appropriate age limits because adults overprotect them or do not fully appreciate their capabilities.

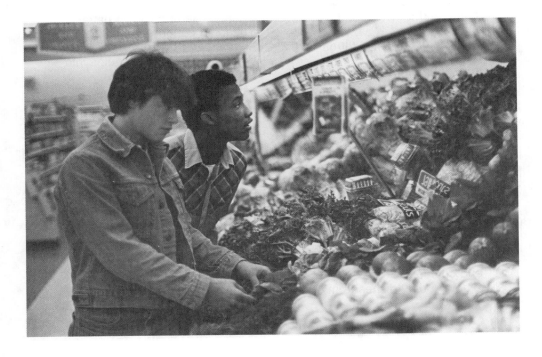

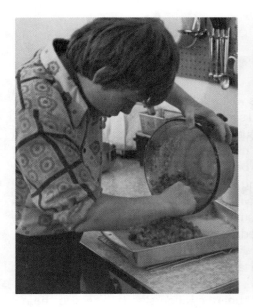
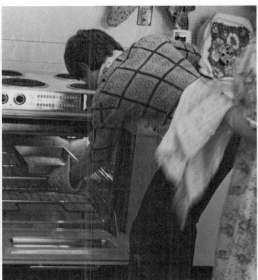

Food management

Helping adults to select food and plan menus

Identifying fruits, vegetables, meats, and dairy products by name and determining their quality

Putting groceries away in proper storage areas

Preparing, labeling, and storing food

Measuring both dry and liquid ingredients

Using such utensils and appliances as can openers, egg beaters, and toasters

Stirring both dry and liquid mixtures

Tossing salads

Slicing vegetables and meats

Mixing cake and cookie batter

Kneading dough and making homemade bread

Pouring hot and cold liquids into cups, glasses or bowls

Labeling food for the freezer or refrigerator

Placing leftovers in storage containers

Wrapping sandwiches for a picnic or lunchbox

Clean-up

Cleaning cutting boards and counters

Removing dirty dishes from the table

Washing, drying, and putting away dishes, pots, pans, and utensils

Scouring sinks and cleaning

Managing a food budget

Using an effective, efficient system of identifying, folding, and storing currency in a wallet

Purchasing, with a specific amount of money, refreshments for a party for two or three friends

Examining foods in different-sized packages and deciding which package is most economical and best suits family needs

Identifying coins and making change

Choice and care of clothing

Planning and selecting a wardrobe

Exploring how fabrics change when treated with heat, water, or chemicals

Discussing the appropriateness of clothing in relation to activities (dress clothes versus play clothes) and seasons

Choosing matching accessories and jewelry

Folding clothes

Recognizing when clothes are dirty and placing them in the hamper

Knowing which clothes can be washed and which need to be dry cleaned

Polishing shoes and recognizing when they need new heels

Using a clothes washer and dryer

Adjusting the temperature setting on an iron and ironing clothes

Putting clothes on hangers

Labeling and storing clothes

Distinguishing similar garments by their unique aspects (buttons, shape of collars, texture)

Labeling clothes that may be worn together, according to their colors and patterns

Folding and storing clothes in dresser drawers or hanging them in a closet

Household maintenance

Selecting tools and cleaning agents

Planning chores on a regular basis

Discussing the importance of cleaning and organizing a room on a scheduled basis

Making needed repairs

Cleaning

Learning to dust and polish

Learning to sweep, mop, and vacuum floors

Learning to clean appliances

Deciding on appropriate cleaning apparatus and materials when presented with a task

Learning to move furniture for cleaning and replacing it in its original position

Learning to wash windows

Differentiating among various cleaning and dusting agents and knowing safety rules to exercise when using them

Preparing the vacuum cleaner for use, including changing the bag, cleaning the receptacle and plugging the cord into the wall outlet

Storage

Knowing how and where to store toys and books when not in use

Learning to organize, store, and locate cleaning aids and tools,

cooking utensils, appliances, and other commonly used items so that they are easily accessible

Money management

Discussing the value of budgeting money

Planning ways to budget

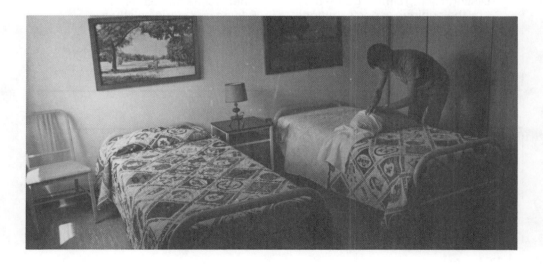

COMMUNICATION

The development of speech and language follows the same pattern for sighted and for blind and visually impaired children. However, children who have had little or no useful vision since birth may have difficulties in acquiring effective communication skills. These include both verbal communication, in which words are used to express thoughts and make one's needs and desires known, and non-verbal communication, in which meaning is conveyed by facial expressions, gestures, and body positions. The child should be encouraged to use both verbal and nonverbal communication skills to request objects and information about people and events, to share, to pretend, and to express emotions.

Verbal communication

Children learn verbal communication, or language, through the association of words with events or objects that are meaningful to them. Language is a highly complex skill that consists of three dimensions: content, structure, and function. With very young children, the function and content of language are the primary focuses of training.

Of the three dimensions of verbal language just noted, it is the content of the language of blind and visually impaired children that will differ most from that of sighted children. Many of the concepts and early vocabulary of sighted children are based on objects and events that are experienced visually.

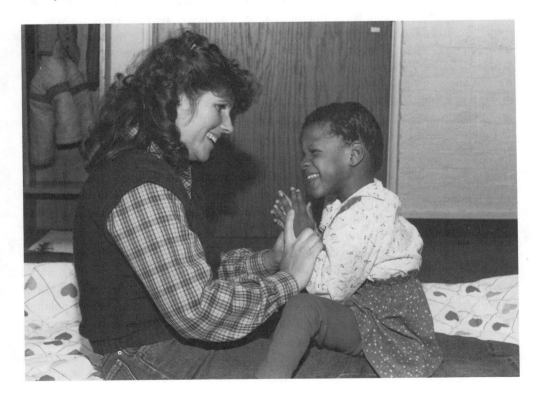

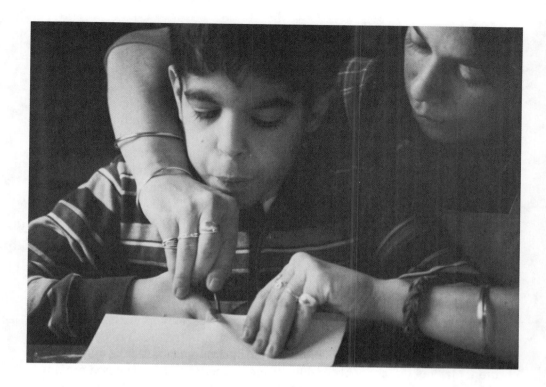

Concepts of objects are especially important to the development of the content or meaning of language. Sighted children learn to associate names with objects as they move toward them, examine them closely, and observe their characteristics; thus, they combine visual, auditory, and tactile impressions to form stable images of objects and people. Very young blind or visually impaired children need encouragement, at the crawling and early walking stages, to explore and re-explore objects and people in the home while the adults help them associate the names of objects with how they feel, sound, and smell, and what they do. In going through these motions on a day-to-day basis, young visually impaired children are encouraged to be aware of their environment.

To ensure that the words that blind and visually impaired children acquire have clear and accurate reference, adults must show and encourage the children to experience what is going on in the environment; for example, children should hear, locate, and feel a ringing telephone; pick it up; listen; and respond. Language training is most effective when it occurs within a context that is meaningful and interesting to children.

Adults can help visually impaired and blind children develop associations between words and objects or actions and learn about the environment in concrete, meaningful ways by involving them in household activities, naming objects, and talking about actions while encouraging the children to be involved in the events. In this way, children acquire the vocabulary that sighted children pick up by repeated visual observation and verification as well as participation.

The emergence of language and the development of thought processes go hand in hand in early childhood. Therefore, it is crucial for very young blind or visually impaired children to gather information about persons, objects, and activities in the environment through direct hands-on experiences. By exploring with all their remaining senses, including the "kinesthetic" sense (muscular activity), these children develop strategies for interpreting and relating to the environment and solving problems while building language skills. This activity establishes a foundation for the performance of more complex intellectual tasks. For example, when introducing a new toy to a child, the adult needs to help the child exploit its possibilities (what it does, what can be done to it, what it is for, and so forth). Otherwise, the child may acquire a vocabulary that has little real meaning and will appear to know more about what is happening in the world than she really does.

Nonverbal communication

Many nonverbal gestures and movements, so common in everyday conversation, are learned by sighted children through observation and imitation. Blind or visually impaired children require specific instruction to acquire these socially meaningful behaviors. Young children should be taught such gestures as reaching, pointing, beckoning, and waving. Older children should feel the motions that the adult is making. Model the movements on a soft cloth doll or floppy stuffed animal, and then move the child's body or hands in the appropriate patterns. Positive feedback about the appropriateness of gestures and motions will encourage children to continue to try to express themselves through gestures and movements.

Smiling, laughing, and frowning come naturally to blind and visually impaired children as well as sighted children early in life. However, they require more conscious efforts by older visually impaired children and adults. The reinforcement of these expressions and recognition of them as ways of communicating feelings are important. Again, positive feedback and consistent encouragement will go a long way toward helping blind and visually impaired children to incorporate these expressions into their everyday patterns of expression.

Listening and comprehending

Listening—attending to auditory stimulation—and comprehending verbal language are vital skills that blind and visually impaired children must develop. Young blind and visually impaired children need to discriminate meaningful sounds in the environment, to interpret these sounds, and to associate them with their sources. They learn to associate sounds with persons, actions, and objects by repeated, concrete, and meaningful experiences that integrate sound, touch, smell, and movement into stable mental references.

Adults can begin to stimulate the blind or visually impaired infant's sense of hearing soon after birth by eliminating unnecessary or distracting noises from the environment so the infant is not overwhelmed or distracted from distinguishing meaningful sounds. They should speak clearly and communicate love while handling, feeding, or holding the infant.

Sighted infants reach out for objects after experiencing them through touch, sound, and sight. Visually impaired and blind infants reach out for things once they know that the objects exist by associating them with their sounds. Adults can facilitate this process by making sure that playthings have a distinctive sound (such as a musical stuffed or mechanical toy) and by gradually encouraging the infants to reach for and identify favorite toys by their sounds (this usually begins toward the end of the first year).

Blind and visually impaired children also need to learn to localize sound. Adults can play "listening games" with toddlers, shaking favorite toys in front of, in back of, and to the side of the child's head and helping the child to turn toward the sound if he does not do so independently. When the child is ready, adults can encourage him to move toward the sound of a voice and sound-producing toys from increasing distances by first providing a constant source of sound and then intermittent sounds, gradually diminishing the length of time of the cue and increasing time between cues.

Once children are able to locate a stationary, direct, and constant source of sound, adults can introduce play activities that involve the tracking or tracing of sounds. Have the child follow your voice, your steps as you march, or a sound-producing toy. At first, provide constant sound cues, then progress to tracking intermittent sound cues. Vary the sound cues by initially using familiar and easily heard sounds, progressing to less familiar and quieter sounds. All such activities should first be introduced in quiet, familiar, and obstruction-free areas in which the child feels comfortable and secure.

Listening skills are essential to blind and visually impaired children who are of school age. Through listening, the child stores information. It is a technique useful for comprehending taped materials. Safe mobility and social awareness are heightened by the auditory channel. It is important that systematic instruction in listening and comprehension techniques be provided by a teacher of visually impaired students. The effective usefulness of this training should never be minimized.

Reading readiness

Readiness for reading and writing, two important avenues of communication, involves skills that are developed during the first few years of life. Children who have had the opportunity to explore the environment through touch, sound, smell, and movement; to interact frequently with family members and friends; to move around freely; to experience a variety of situations outside the home; and who have been read to by adults will have the experiential background necessary to begin reading.

"Twin-Vision" books are inkprint with braille overlays that help young children learn that words can be either seen or touched. Putting labels (braille labels for blind children and large-print labels for visually impaired children) on storage shelves for toys and books also will help children learn to associate written symbols with their meanings.

Furthermore, visually impaired children should be taught to recognize and identify letters using large-print letters with high contrast backgrounds. When they are ready to read, the teacher of visually impaired children will help evaluate what type of visual materials and aids will be most suitable for their reading needs.

Children with no useful vision can develop sensitivity in their fingers through a variety of activities, going from gross movements, such as playing with modeling clay, to more refined tasks, such as buttoning and unbuttoning, stringing beads, and lacing or sewing on homemade or commercial cards.

Visually impaired children with vision that is useful for reading benefit most from being encouraged to utilize their vision efficiently and to the maximum extent possible. Adults can make sure that young children are allowed the time to explore people and objects visually at close range, when necessary. They can explore with children, providing information and suggesting further ways of visual inspection. On outings, hikes, or walks, children can be encouraged to talk about what they are seeing.

Multihandicapped visually impaired children face additional difficulties in developing communication skills, depending on the nature of the other disabilities. These children need a great deal of systematic stimulation and intervention on all levels of functioning to learn about themselves and the environment before they express themselves through language. Developmentally delayed blind children go through the same stages of language development as do other visually impaired or sighted children, but they do so more slowly. It is essential for adults to work with a specialist in an infant stimulation program that is designed to meet the specific, complex, and individual needs of these children.

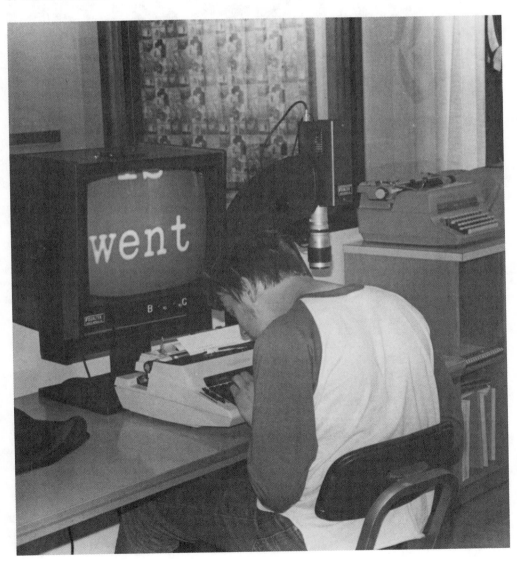

LEARNING THROUGH PLAY

All children learn through play. Infants, toddlers, and school age children alike profit immeasurably from the opportunity to perfect their developing minds and bodies through an infinite variety of activities. Play gives blind and visually impaired children a vital opportunity to practice and integrate all the skills they are striving to master. Understanding objects, interacting with other children, learning to move in space and time, gaining awareness of the body, developing large and small muscles through move-

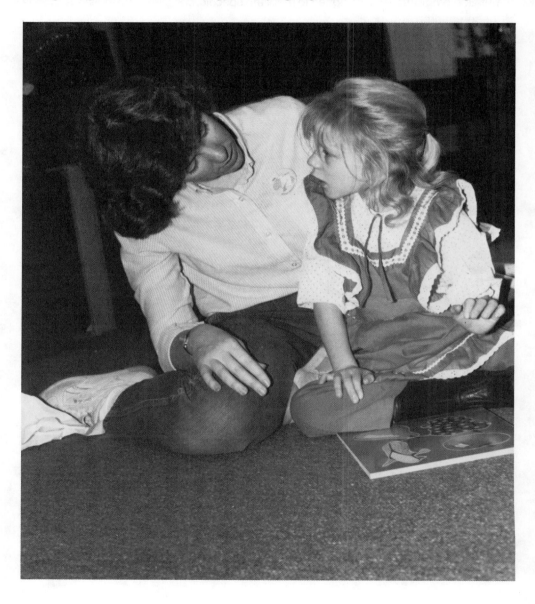

ment, and expressing thoughts, feelings, and ideas can be facilitated through play activities. Play-acting (such as "playing house" or "playing fireman") helps children to develop imagination, understanding, and language as well as to refine thought.

Play starts in infancy when infants randomly, then deliberately, engage in pleasurable activities. It assists them to become familiar with their bodies and the world around them. Adults can do a great deal to help children enjoy themselves and develop during these early months by providing appropriate stimulation. Two such sources of stimulation are mobiles and rattles.

A mobile for the crib of a blind or visually impaired infant should be made of noisy objects, such as small balls with bells inside and, in the case of visually impaired infants, brightly colored objects, such as plastic disks, beads, and keys. The mobile should be strung across the crib close enough to the child's body that he or she will accidentally encounter the objects while moving arms and legs. Rattles can be constructed by filling small cardboard or plastic boxes with beans, rice, or popcorn, and covering them with materials of different textures.

The toddler stage is a time for moving around and "getting into things"— discovering the functions of objects and the limits of what one can do with one's body, with other people, and with objects. Some of the many simple activities enjoyed by toddlers are: 1) fitting pots and pans into each other and finding out how much noise can be made with them, 2) banging spoons against objects and inserting them into boxes, and 3) discovering the function of toys with graduated sizes (such as stacking rings or barrels that fit into each other). These activities should be introduced to toddlers and explored with them.

At the preschool stage, it is crucial to provide visually impaired and blind children with opportunities for imaginative, expressive play. Two such examples are *playing with water*, in which the adult and child explore what can be done with many types of containers in the water (pouring, spilling, splashing, and so forth) and *playing with blocks*, in which the adult and child explore various concepts by building houses, walls, roads, and bridges.

In the elementary school years, blind and visually impaired children enjoy, along with peers, games that are structured and rule-oriented (at this age, children are defining themselves as parts of a social system). Adults can help by making sure that the children have plenty of opportunities to socialize and play with other children and by reinforcing skills by playing board games, catch, and word games with them.

Adolescents need the opportunity to expand their skills, test their limits, and enjoy socializing by choosing from a wide variety of recreational activities, such as skiing, swimming, special-interest clubs, and hiking.

LOW-VISION DEVICES

Some children easily incorporate prescribed optical devices into their lives, while others refuse to use them except under certain conditions. It is important to remember that optical devices do not restore or give normal vision to visually impaired children. They do, however, help children to maximize their use of vision to perform certain tasks. Parents must carefully examine their own reactions to and feelings about optical devices before they can support the child's use of these devices. Young children seem to accept the use of devices more readily if the devices are presented in a positive and supportive manner, and preschoolers may enjoy playing with toy magnifiers and telescopes. If these devices are available and seem to have a purpose, the children may later accept them more readily for academic and mobility purposes if they have played with and used them earlier.

It is important that children incorporate devices into their learning styles as early as possible so the devices are part of their pattern of learning. Behaviors that have always been a part of a child's pattern are more beneficial than those that are added later to the learner's environment or learning style. Also, the child will benefit from the longer use of the devices.

Adults who present devices to visually impaired children should understand how the specific devices can be best used and believe in the benefits that can be derived from their efficient use. Optical devices can be used in a variety of settings. For example, binoculars or monoculars can be used at a ball game, the theater, or the circus and magnifiers help children to read restaurant menus independently.

Devices are conspicuous and identify the user as visually impaired only in certain circumstances. Although visually impaired children, especially adolescents, may be self-conscious and dread being different from their peers, they must weigh their need to belong against the benefits to be derived from using optical devices. Some children consider their identification as visually impaired to be a benefit because "passing" as a sighted person can create frustrations or make it more difficult to ask for assistance.

It should be pointed out, however, that the use of optical devices can cause children to think that they should no longer ask for assistance. This is not the case. Devices, when properly used, have their restrictive qualities; a small field of view for high-power monoculars or a short focal length for strong spectacle lenses may result in a slower, though independent, reading speed. Therefore, children will still need help from others, although to a lesser extent. They must come to understand that optical devices are just another set of tools that are used in conjunction with recordings, readers, and other technological devices.

When children come into contact with others who question the use of devices, they may feel self-conscious. It is recommended that children be taught to respond to such questions by explaining the reason for the devices and how they function. Role playing may be helpful in preparing children for such situations. It may also be suggested that children demonstrate devices to their classmates at sharing time.

Older children, even those who earlier readily accepted devices, may suddenly reject even the use of glasses. A need for peer acceptance and conformity, particularly during adolescence, should be seen as a normal aspect of psychosocial development. Adolescence is a difficult time for all; calling attention to one's impairment may seem too high a price if adolescents fear it will "cost" them their social status. During this crucial time, adults should continue to encourage adolescents to use devices and help them to see that additional independence through increased visual input is part of a positive self-identity. After this period, young adults generally will reaccept devices if they are truly useful and beneficial.

Parents may wish to let their children experiment with a variety of hand-held magnifiers or talk about the changes that occur when distances are changed, the power of the magnification increased, and so forth. They can provide their children with experiences in which the children can try out devices (if so prescribed); for instance, reading bus and store signs, and attending sports events, help them role play potentially positive or negative situations, and teach them to speak for themselves when questions arise.

Prosthetic eyes. Children of all ages should learn to take care of their false eyes and to feel comfortable about them. A young child may take part in cleansing them by doing simple tasks even before he is ready to take full responsibility for them. A school-age child may be ready to learn to insert the eye or eyes and to clean the facial area around the eye. Not only is the child learning to take care of the prosthesis as part of a daily grooming routine, but he is learning to assume responsibility, which helps the child feel more capable of handling future situations, such as excessive tearing while at school, which may necessitate the removal, cleaning, and reinsertion of the prosthetic eye.

The classroom teacher should be prepared in advance about the care of prosthetic eyes by the parent or teacher of visually impaired children. The child should be advised not to pop the eye out in class just to get attention. The teacher should determine the cause of this behavior and try to eliminate it, initiating a behavioral management system, if necessary.

SEX EDUCATION

It is often assumed that blind and visually impaired students are receiving age-appropriate sex education, but they usually are not. With the present openness about information, there should be no reason why any group of students should suffer anxiety, fear, or ignorance about their sexual desires or functions. In addition, young women need basic information and direct instruction in gynecological problems and body hygiene. Both young men and women should be prepared for changes that they will experience with the coming of puberty.

Many topics related to sex should be discussed with visually impaired children and their parents, guardians and sex education teachers. It is essential that these adults communicate with each other to be sure that all relevant topics are discussed with and learned by the child. Some topics include physical differences, changes at puberty, intercourse, reproduction, pregnancy cycle, childbirth, teen pregnancies, sexually transmitted diseases, sexual feelings and attractions, communicating with members of the opposite sex, sexual decision-making, homosexuality, values, media and sex, peer pressure, masturbation, teenage marriages, love relationships, commitments, family planning, contraception methods, gynecological examinations, abortion, rape, and sexual abuse.

The body

Blind and visually impaired children should be given the opportunity to learn about changes that occur in the bodies of both males and females during puberty, including the growth of body hair and breasts and increased genital sensations, and to become familiar with the physical structures of adult male and female forms. Such opportunities are often, but not always, best experienced at home under the guidance of caring and open parents or guardians. In addition, these children should be given the same sex education courses as their sighted peers even though their instruction requires tactile exploration because they cannot learn from visual observation. Despite the cultural, religious, and social taboos against touching, exceptions must be made for blind and visually impaired children in these courses so they will be able to gain a realistic understanding of the physical differences and similarities of the male and female forms. In this regard, realistic, commercially available models and live models should be considered as learning aids.

Vocabulary. The correct terms for various parts of the body and for sexual activities should be explained, and the meaning of derogatory implications of slang terms, as well as the social conditions in which they are used, should be understood. Some young men and women may find such language offensive, but some may need to be made aware that others do not appreciate hearing slang sexual terms.

Menstruation

Instruction about menstruation should begin before a girl's first menarche, when obvious bodily changes—the development of breasts and the growth of underarm and pubic hair— are rapidly occurring with the onset of puberty. The girl and her parents should plan for her first menstrual period with an open attitude, which will later typify the directness with which they will discuss all sexual questions and concerns. Classroom discussion, although less personal, can be effective and can help girls realize that menstruation is a natural phenomenon that all women experience.

In preparation for the first menstrual period, parents may wish to help their daughters prepare a kit to be placed in the school locker. The kit for school may include sanitary napkins, a washcloth and small towel, soap, paper bags for disposal of the napkin, and a clean pair of panties. Sanitary napkins should also be stored in the bathroom or bedroom.

Blind girls must learn to open the sanitary napkin box and learn why a napkin is used. They must be taught how to place the adhesive pad, identify the right and wrong sides, peel off the paper strip, center and secure the pad on the panty, and dispose of the soiled napkin at home or in a public bathroom. Various sizes of sanitary napkins should be introduced with appropriate accompanying explanations.

Blind girls also need to know how to recognize that the menstrual period has begun and learn to determine how often they need to change sanitary napkins or tampons. Because they cannot check by sight to verify the start and flow of menstruation, they must therefore feel, touch, and possibly smell the menstrual discharge. In addition, they must become aware of the internal and physical sensations at the onset of menstruation and know what actually is happening to the body as well as why it is happening.

Both blind and visually impaired girls must also learn to wash soiled clothing and bedding. They should be aware that bedding must be removed immediately and soaked in cold water to avoid staining. Menstrual discharge has an odor that is readily identifiable and requires immediate attention.

There is nothing more irregular than the "regular" menstrual cycle. When a girl first begins to menstruate, ovulation often does not occur on a regular basis. Therefore, the teenager should become aware of those factors that might lead her to expect her next menstrual period. Later, ovulation generally becomes more regular. With a longer time between periods, the girl is building up the excess lining of the uterus, so when discharge begins, it may appear profuse. When her first cycle begins, she should be encouraged to change sanitary napkins at frequent and regular intervals, determined, in part, by her rate of flow; she may need help in determining the appropriate schedule.

Visually impaired teenagers should receive all the consumer information on how to select and buy sanitary napkins (or tampons) and where they are located in stores and public restrooms. The possible dangers in using tampons should be discussed with their mothers and gynecologists, as well as the comparative benefits and uses of napkins versus tampons. When tampons are going to be used, their insertion, removal, and disposal must be thoroughly explained and practiced.

Learning how to purchase a napkin from a public restroom dispenser involves locating and recognizing a napkin dispenser, inserting the coins, turning the handle, and obtaining the boxed napkin. Since the napkin may not have an adhesive backing, the girl must learn how to use a pad with pins. She must learn to ask if her clothing is spotted and know how to wash out spots without getting the entire piece of clothing wet. Most frequently, she can get help from a teacher or friend. Since some public restrooms may not have a napkin dispenser, or it may be impossible to locate, the girl must also know how to use toilet paper or paper towels until she can obtain a sanitary napkin or tampon.

Visiting the gynecologist. Blind and visually impaired girls should be informed about all the aspects of an impending examination. When they arrive at the gynecologist's office, the doctor or nurse should familiarize them with the examination table and instruments, tell them what to expect during the examination, and help them to feel comfortable about discussing menstrual problems, symptoms, and concerns.

Masturbation

It is a common phenomenon for both males and females to experiment with and practice masturbation. However, young visually impaired and blind youngsters should be made aware of their families' and society's cultural and religious beliefs about masturbation and that masturbation activities should be performed in private. Young men should be taught about the phenomenon of wet dreams.

Dating

Dating behaviors and customs should be discussed. It is often helpful to role play such situations as asking someone out on a date. In addition, alternative transportation methods associated with dating should be explored, including double dating and the use of public transportation or cab services. Blind and visually impaired adolescents should be encouraged to discuss their dating experiences and feelings with adult role models.

Genetic Counseling

Blind and visually impaired adolescents have concerns about whether their handicapping condition is hereditary and whether they should plan to have children. They should be told about the role and activities of genetic counselors and how they might contact these counselors if they so chose. It should be made clear that genetic counselors do not make recommendations regarding childbearing but merely analyze genetic facts and present information on the percentage of chance that the impairment is likely to be passed on to offspring.

Teachers, paraprofessionals, and other adults who work with blind and visually impaired children in matters associated with sex education should learn about their employer's (school or agency) policies about sex education and about parents' attitudes toward it. Because sex education is a delicate and even volatile subject, those who teach it should take appropriate precautions to safeguard themselves from possible disciplinary actions.

Part II
ORIENTATION AND MOBILITY

INTRODUCTION

Independent mobility is a basic freedom that most people take for granted. However, the lack of motivation, uncertainty, and even fear of movement can seriously affect the future independence of blind and visually impaired children. From the start, the mobility of visually impaired and blind children develops at a slower rate than that of sighted children. Because blind and visually impaired children cannot see objects at a distance, they are not as motivated as are sighted children to move toward people and objects or to explore in the environment; thus, they are deprived of early experiences that lead to learning. Guidance and stimulation by parents, teachers, and other concerned adults can provide these children with opportunities to explore and learn.

Blind and visually impaired children need to be actively involved in all the routines of daily life so they can learn and apply the skills they must have to travel independently. Therefore, adults should take every opportunity to expand the child's understanding of the environment, provide opportunities to develop independent mobility, and encourage the application of learned skills. Furthermore, children who need to learn sensory and cane skills for safe and independent travel must receive specialized instruction from orientation and mobility instructors. The freedom of choice that independent mobility allows cannot be duplicated.

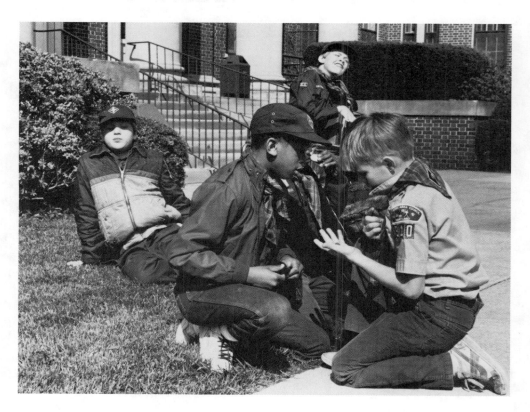

CONCEPTS

Orientation and mobility

Orientation is the ability to become familiar with an unknown environment. Sighted children learn about and feel comfortable with their environments by using their vision, as well as their other senses. They become aware of new physical surroundings within a matter of seconds. But blind and visually impaired children need to explore, carefully and systematically, new surroundings using their sensory systems. The effective utilization of all the remaining senses requires practice and feedback that confirms or corrects the children's interpretations. As they grow older, blind and visually impaired children will have an increased need to orient themselves to unfamiliar environments. Learning to use the remaining senses, incorporating concepts that are inherent to environments, and structuring organizational procedures are integral components of meaningful orientation.

Children should be encouraged to explore their environments, starting with their cribs, rooms, and other parts of their homes and to learn the appropriate labels for objects, textures, colors, temperatures, sounds, and so forth. Although it is possible to be mobile in unfamiliar areas, mobility is easier and movement more efficient when one is familiar with one's surroundings. Therefore, blind and visually impaired children need to learn how to familiarize—orient—themselves to ever-changing environments.

Mobility is the act of moving in space. Independent mobility allows one the freedom to come and go as one chooses.

When sighted children are stimulated by stationary or moving objects and want to make contact with them, they reach out and try to creep, crawl, walk, or run to them. Visually impaired and blind children should be provided with meaningful stimulation so they are motivated to move about independently. One such source of stimulation is tactually pleasing, sound-producing, and colorful toys, which should first be presented and then pulled beyond reach while still producing sound, so a child will learn to reach for the object. The child must know and like the toy and associate it with its sound before he or she will move toward it. Therefore, the toy should not be placed at a distance from the child until he or she has had a chance to explore it tactually and, if possible, visually.

Direct intervention may be required before blind and visually impaired children can creep, crawl, walk, run, or complete other physical actions. The children should be encouraged to explore and move about, while an adult explains and provides appropriate feedback, and the environments in which they travel should gradually increase in size and variety.

Visually impaired and blind children must be provided with a wealth of sensory experiences and the opportunity to explore independently with all their remaining senses, including vision. They cannot do so if they are physically led through life. Well-meaning adults may attempt to protect them from the hazards of the environment by offering too much assistance or by excluding them from experiences that sighted

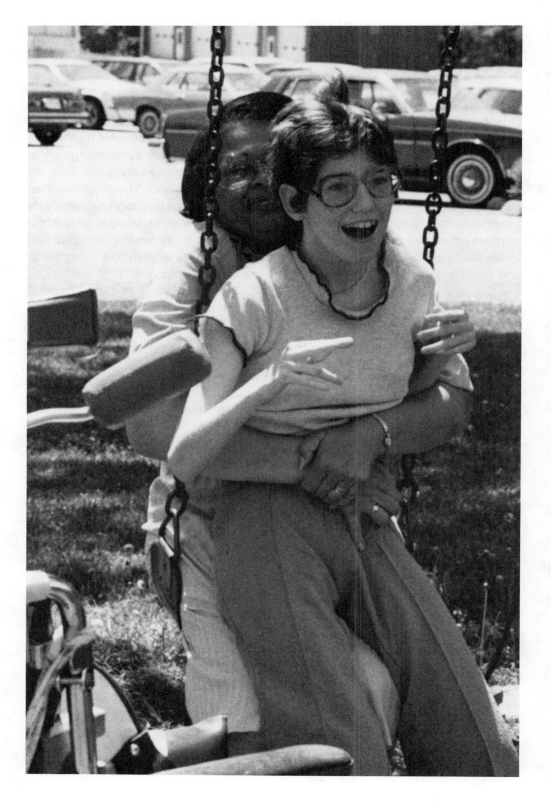

children normally encounter. Overprotection makes children passive and dependent and stifles their natural curiosity. If they are deprived of opportunities to explore and move, they will lack the experiences necessary for learning concepts and obtaining meaningful information about their environments.

Awareness of the body

The ability of visually impaired and blind children to learn about the outside world and how to interact with it depends first on how well they understand and can relate to their bodies. Knowing the names, movements, and functions of parts of the body and how these parts relate to each other and to the environment enhances the child's ability to move independently.

Games such as "Touch your—" help children to identify parts of their bodies. However, just pointing to a spot on an arm or thigh is not sufficient. Rather, children should learn where a body part begins and ends, how it moves and in which directions, and what its purposes are. Such knowledge can facilitate their learning other concepts and movements.

After children have learned to identify the parts of their bodies, they should be able to transfer this knowledge to the bodies of family members, dolls and other toys, and animals. Adults should then reinforce this knowledge while giving directions in different situations.

Children who have enough vision can play with pictures and body puzzles, naming and assembling the different body parts. They can tell an adult the names of various parts and describe the location of these parts on the body. The adult can ask them to place their side against the wall, to lie flat on their back, and so on. "Simon Says" is an enjoyable way of teaching children how to place parts of their bodies in different positions. (For instance, "Simon says, 'Place your side against the wall'").

To help children understand how body parts move and function in relation to one another, an adult can demonstrate such movements as bending, twisting, rotating, lifting, and turning and then ask the child to identify and move the parts of the body that are involved. Children with usable vision should be encouraged to imitate the adults' movements while applying the correct terminology.

Spatial concepts

Spatial concepts, such as over, under, up, down, side, and back, should be incorporated routinely into daily learning activities. Children can be taught to follow directions, such as bending, hopping, turning to the right, moving forward, taking three steps to the left, and stepping two to the right.

Terms of laterality, such as left and right, should be introduced in relation to the child's body movements and then to objects and other persons. Although concepts of laterality are often difficult to master and are learned later than spatial concepts, adults should use the terms with young children in preparation for direction instruction in these concepts. In teaching laterality, the adult should place objects (rubber bands, watches, rings, etc.) on one side of the child's body and ask the child to identify which side they are on. After the child has learned to identify one side, the adult should switch the objects to the other side and repeat the procedure. Next, mixed directions, such as "Place the ring on your right thumb and the watch on your left wrist" should be given.

Children need to understand that their right and left sides remain constant but, depending on which way they are facing, someone or something can be to their right or left. This concept can be introduced by having children identify which side of their body is closest to an object or person. After they have mastered this ability, the adult can move on to discussing the sides of other individuals when they are facing the same direction. Stand behind the child, facing the child's back while she holds your arm. Then move in front of and face the child and demonstrate how your right hand has now moved to the child's left. Wear a watch, rubber band, or ring consistently on one hand so the child will have a tangible object to confirm the change in positions. Move in various positions in relation to the child and ask her to locate your right arm, left shoulder, and so forth. Then conduct similar activities using objects. Reverse the process so that you remain constant and the child moves around you. Have the child use toys and identify their positions in relation to each other.

Directionality

If children are to move and function successfully in the environment, they must learn the meaning of such abstract directional concepts as up/down, in/out and above/below. They begin to do so by using their body as a reference system and moving the various parts in relation to each other by placing their bodies in various positions in relation to objects, and by manipulating objects in relation to each other.

To teach the concept of inside, place the child *inside* a box large enough for comfort and small enough so he can easily reach the top, bottom, and all four sides without moving the body. Have the child feel all the inside sides of the box and then tap the *inside* of the box. Hold a musical toy outside the box and ask the child to reach for it, take, and place it *inside* the box. Once the child has mastered the concept of inside, progress to a smaller box and have the child place objects *inside* and *outside* the box on command. Whenever possible, incorporate these concepts into activities that the child enjoys, such as putting toys inside a toy box and a wagon inside the garage. Avoid words and phrases such as "here" or "over there" because these words will have no meaning for a child who cannot see which way you are facing or pointing.

All the concepts that are taught should have an immediate and practical application. Because many blind children have difficulty transferring newly learned concepts to situations that were not involved in the learning process, it is important to have them apply what they learn to functional and practical tasks in many different settings.

Time and distance

Time and distance are difficult concepts for blind and visually impaired children to learn. Because they must estimate and project beyond their bodies to understand these concepts, they must be frequently exposed to these concepts, discuss them, and receive reinforcement in using them.

These concepts may be introduced by providing guidelines about what happens at different times of the day and talking about what happened yesterday, what is happening today, what will occur tomorrow. Children can be taught to estimate the length of a second, five minutes, and an hour and use an auditory timer or alarm clock to reinforce what they learn. Adults should discuss how much time it takes to dress in the morning, eat a meal, walk to a friend's house and so forth and have the child estimate how long it will take to do routine daily activities by reading a watch, doing the activity, and then checking the time it took to do so.

To help the child understand distance, invent games and activities that involve short lengths, such as an inch, a foot, or a yard. Measure parts of the child's body to use as reference points and then measure the child's stride and the distances between permanently placed objects with which she is familiar. The child can then estimate how many feet she is from different objects in the room. Help the child use a modified rule or yardstick with tactile markings to measure and confirm distances. While taking the child for walks or drives, indicate the distance you have traveled and the time it took to get to a place.

North, south, east, and west

The concepts of north, south, east, west and their combinations are often difficult to learn. They should not be introduced until the child has mastered the basic concepts of space and directionality. Begin with a known room where the child is familiar with the four different walls and can identify each correctly. Label these north, south, east, and west. Teach the child to make accurate turns by facing each wall. Next, give the child increasingly difficult sequences of routes, such as "You are facing north, take three steps and turn west" and verbalize which way he will be turning and repeat the directions before proceeding. Gradually introduce outside route reversals and alternate routes. The child should learn to identify important landmarks in order to verify the direction. Adults must always give accurate and complete information to avoid confusing the blind or visually impaired child.

AWARENESS OF THE ENVIRONMENT

Knowledge of objects and events beyond the familiar boundaries of home and family is essential to a child's growth as a whole person. There is a limit to how much of the outside world can and should be brought to the child. Thus, the child needs to learn about the world through experiences in many different environments.

Listen with the child to the morning sounds around the house and school. Help the child name the sources and imitate the sounds. Encourage the child to verbalize her awareness of familiar or newly learned sounds, such as a bird singing, toast popping from the toaster, or a window rattling in the wind. On a hike or walk, name the things you touch in the environment—a stone, a rail, grass, flowers, trees, the sidewalk, a coat, or a friend's hand. Prepare a lunch or school snack with the child's help, describing each step of the preparation so the child will identify the sounds that go with the actions (for example, the knife chopping the celery for tuna salad or the refrigerator door opening and closing). Talk about the various types of clues to look for in identifying actions, odors and sounds.

Take the child to the grocery store to help you find food items and name them. Help the child classify the items (dairy, vegetables, canned food, etc.). Observe the temperatures near the refrigerator and freezer sections and ask the child to identify the foods that need cold storage. The youngster should participate in every step, feeling and smelling foods, identifying them, learning how to determine their quality, what they are used for, and how much they cost. At home, the child can help put the groceries away so he will learn how food is stored. Also discuss how various foods are prepared and involve the child in preparing them. When the child has the appropriate skills, he can go to the local store and make purchases independently, take and pick up clothes from the dry cleaners, and do similar errands.

Integration of self and objects in space

Children need to understand how their relationships to objects change as they move through an environment. To teach this concept, have the child back against the wall and then step forward. Ask where the wall is and whether the child can reach and touch it. Then have the child move farther away from the wall until it cannot be reached. What has moved, the child or the wall? Encourage the child to try different ways of moving away from as well as toward the wall. Have the child move toward a radio across the room, telling you where it is in relation to herself and to other objects in the room. Have the child change position in relation to a constant sound source, such as a radio, and then change the radio's position in relation to other objects in the room. The child should analyze the changes and later move to them to verify her conclusions.

Later, try a more advanced training activity. Using a square or rectangular block of a neighborhood, walk along one street, identifying significant landmarks until you arrive at a corner. Turn onto a new street and continue around the four sides of the block, pausing to note landmarks such as neighbors' homes, a store, a vacant lot, or the turns onto new streets. Ask the child to identify the shape or geometric form you

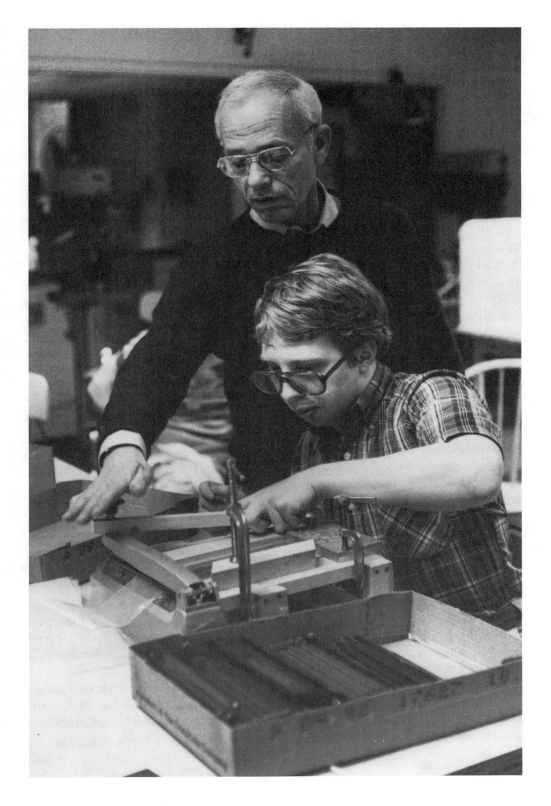

walked (square or rectangle). Ask for other examples of the shape, assuming, of course, that you provided numerous opportunities for the child to develop stable concepts of shapes. Have the child describe where he is in relation to the starting point and significant landmarks and how to get to specific streets and landmarks in the block, using the longest and shortest routes. Another day, walk the opposite way around the same block and see if the child can tell you the similarities and differences of the two routes. The child should take notice of the surroundings as you walk and listen to and separate the sounds of vehicles in motion and idling traffic sounds and patterns. Continue this process when you walk with the child to and from friends' homes, the park, or local stores. Take turns with the child in identifying the sound of a car or other vehicle and the way it is moving (left to right or north to south). Have a contest to see who can hear the vehicles coming first. Can the child tell if it is a car, a truck, or a bus?

The child should practice telling you when cars are stopping and have stopped at a red light and when they begin to move again after the light changes to green. Talk about which way the cars are moving and when pedestrians can cross the street. How many ways can the cars go? Where do the streets meet? Discuss the types and shapes of intersections. Name a busy road and a quiet street; walk along them and compare the sounds and number of cars you hear along the way. Listen to the noises of motors, brakes, horns, and the sounds of traffic stopping and starting. Help the child relax as you walk in busy areas. Let the child know that the sounds she hears will help her learn how to cross streets safely.

Landmarks and clues

A **landmark** is any familiar, stationary, permanent object that the child recognizes and therefore can serve as a clue to his location. Some examples include a water cooler, a door, a teacher's desk, a mailbox, or the only traffic-light-controlled intersection in the area.

A **clue** is any recognizable sensory cue that helps the child identify her position in the environment. It need not be stationary or permanent. It may be the smell of a bakery or shoe store, the sounds from a pet store or gas station, a driveway ramp, a draft from an open lot or alley between store fronts, or the sounds of traffic stopping at a stop sign.

In games of tag, a sound-producing object, such as an air conditioner or radio, might be a temporary landmark, whereas traffic or construction sounds might be a directional clue. On a walk through the neighborhood, point out tactual, olfactory, auditory, and (if the child has useful vision) visual landmarks; on the return trip, have the child indicate the clues and landmarks. Indoors, first show the child the door as a landmark, then have the child explore the walls of the room and note where objects are placed. The child should be aware of the location of objects in relation to the landmark and be able to make trips to the objects, first from the door, then from other parts of the room.

Once children learn how to identify and orient themselves, take them to new places and encourage them to explore their surroundings in a systematic manner. In all these instances, provide feedback on the accuracy of their orientation, identification of objects, and determination of reliable landmarks.

SENSORY TRAINING

It is through the use of the five senses that all people learn about and perceive the world in which they live. Visually impaired and blind children must learn to use their senses just as sighted children do. The commonly held belief that visually impaired individuals have more acute senses than sighted individuals is a fallacy. For visually impaired or blind children to use their senses efficiently and accurately, they must be encouraged to utilize input from all the senses (including any vision); provided with appropriate feedback; taught how to apply the senses to gain, integrate, and accurately interpret information for specific tasks; and taught to be flexible in and feel confident about using the senses.

Vision. Regardless of how little light perception (the ability to distinguish light from dark) or light projection (the ability to determine the source of light) children have and how poor their visual acuity or how small their visual field, they should be encouraged to use their sight. With appropriate intervention, they can learn to use their remaining sight in daily activities. Keep in mind that seeing is a learned activity and that, without proper encouragement, children will not learn to use their remaining sight to their best advantage.

Hearing. The specific aspects or skills of hearing that blind and visually impaired children need to develop include recognizing, identifying, locating, selecting, tracking, and discriminating sounds. Each skill must be learned in relation to direct, indirect, and reflected sounds. Direct sound is one that travels directly to the listener without traveling through or around objects. Indirect sound is one that travels through or around objects before reaching the listener, such as sounds in a neighboring room. Reflected sounds are those that travel to a barrier, hit, and bounce back to the listener. Reflected sounds are most commonly exemplified by deeply recessed doorways common to shoe stores. Mall sounds travel to the entrance and are reflected back to the listener at the building line. Such reflection changes the quality of the sound and makes it echo-like.

The senses of smell, taste, and touch also should be developed. For example, aromas and their sources in various settings should be identified; foods that are salty, sweet, bitter, or spicy should be sampled; and the entire body should be involved in determining the textures and degree of softness or hardness of objects, gradient changes, and temperature. Be sure the child can recognize danger signs, such as the smell of gas, excessive heat and cold, sour milk and other spoiled foods.

TRAVEL TECHNIQUES AND DEVICES

Blind and visually impaired children, like all children, gradually need to become independent and self-reliant. Parents and other adults who are concerned with safety may be tempted to restrict their children's travel. However, children need to travel, to have experiences related to travel, and to receive specialized training in orientation and mobility techniques. With instruction, children can learn to travel safely and efficiently.

Travel skills include protection techniques, information gathering and planning. One important aid to independent travel is the cane. Parents and other adults can be primary facilitators of a child's understanding of environments, but the teaching of specific travel skills, such as the use of a long cane and crossing streets, should be the responsibility of orientation and mobility specialists.

Dependent travel techniques

Sighted guide — contact technique. This technique involves the use of a sighted person to provide guidance, protection, and information. The child should grip the arm of the sighted person above the wrist or above the elbow (depending on the age and size of the child) so the child is one-half step behind and directly beside the guide. The child can then follow the movements of the guide and anticipate any changes

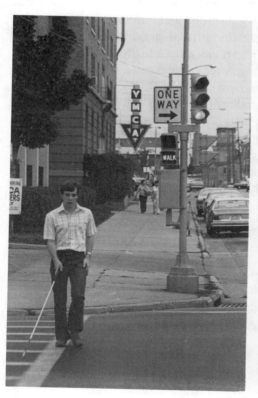
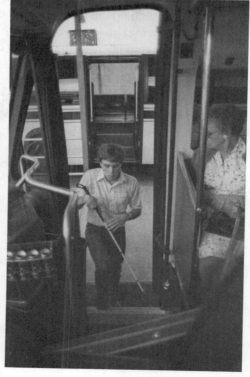

in the path of travel. The guide should tell the child when there are steps, if the steps go up or down, and should stop at the top of the first step to allow the child to pause, feel the edge of the step with her foot, become aligned with the stairs, and grasp the railing. When the guide reaches the landing (top or bottom) of the stairway, he should take one step forward and pause, giving the child a nonverbal signal that they have completed the ascent or descent, allowing the child room to step onto the landing.

The guide should also give appropriate information about doors (whether they open toward or away from the child and if they are on the left or on the right side), narrow passageways, obstacles, and so on. The guide can also help the child locate objects by giving verbal directions, placing his hand on the object, and letting the child's hand slide to it, or placing the child's hand on the object. The guide should be sure that both the guide and the child are holding a railing, when possible, or that the child is on the railing side, when only one railing is available.

Sighted guide—non-contact technique. This technique can be used to give pertinent information about the area, safety considerations, and directions while walking alongside a child. It also can be used to help the child take a seat.

In helping the child take a seat, bring the child to the back of a chair, and have the child extend her free hand to contact it. The child should then trail (maintain contact with) the back, side, and front of the chair while moving to the front. Before sitting, the child should clear the chair (sweep a hand over the seat) to be sure it is free of objects. The child should then place the back of her legs against the edge of the seat and lower herself into the chair. If it is not possible to bring the child to the back of the chair, tell the child what part of the chair she will contact first.

Independent travel techniques

Self-protective techniques. For safety in indoor travel, the child places his arm, bent at an obtuse angle at the elbow, across the upper body with the palm facing outward. The fingers of the protecting arm should extend to align with the opposite shoulder. This position provides a bumper for large above-the-waist objects like walls and doorways. The child can use his free hand for protection from lower obstacles by dropping the arm diagonally downward in front of and away from the body with the palm of the hand turned inward.

Another protective technique is trailing, which should be used only in familiar indoor areas. Using the upper-arm protective method just described with the arm farthest from the wall, the child extends the arm nearest the wall with the elbow straight and the back of the knuckles of the trailing hand gently following the wall. The trailing arm is always kept in front of the body so it can alert the child to doorways, corridors, and other landmarks.

Route following. Independent travel should be encouraged as soon as the child is ready. When the child can travel, she should be expected to do so all the time, taking first simple, then increasingly complex routes. Begin teaching a new route by taking the child along the route, explaining it, and pointing out landmarks. After the child has learned the route to an objective, begin to teach the return route in the same manner. After the child has learned several routes and return routes, have the child begin to reverse the route through his own deductive reasoning. Once the child has learned how to follow routes, verbal directions will be sufficient.

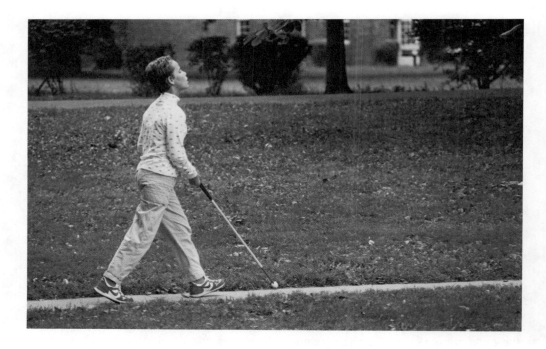

Young blind and visually impaired children should be encouraged to play games that involve following directions. For instance, the child can play "messenger" and bring an important message to a person or place. Tactile versions of games such as Monopoly or Life are excellent for learning to follow directions to destinations, as well as for developing geometric concepts.

When ready, the child can be shown a route to a classroom or to a nearby friend's house. The child should be helped to practice the route until he can travel to the destination safely and independently. Then errands can be run, such as taking milk money to the school office or a teacher, or returning a borrowed object to a next-door neighbor.

Route planning. As their travel skills develop, blind and visually impaired children can be encouraged to plan their own routes. To teach a child how to plan a route, first have the child plan her way around a small obstacle leading to a specific destination, then around increasingly larger obstacles. Once this technique has been mastered, the child should learn to plan increasingly complex routes from room to room in a school or unfamiliar building and to discover alternate routes to the same destination.

Route planning in familiar and eventually unfamiliar locations is easier if the child learns what is necessary to consider in planning a route. Tactile bingo and checkers are useful for developing such route-planning skills as the connection of diagonal corners. Older children may enjoy "store riddles" in which the child plans the move necessary to reach each item you name in a familiar store. After the child becomes confident, you can play the game in new stores, or the child can play "adult" and guide you through the store.

Recovery skills. If a blind child makes a wrong turn and becomes disoriented, he should not be permitted to wander aimlessly, "hoping" to find his way, because such wandering generally creates greater confusion and anxiety. Rather, the child should be prompted to attend to meaningful sensory cues and landmarks that will help identify where he is and what needs to be done to become reoriented.

While walking along a route that a child is attempting to learn, you can help teach the child how to become reoriented through the use of recovery techniques and attention to sensory information and landmarks, and by stressing that recovery skills involve problem-solving and thinking logically. Guide the child's attention to the most useful pieces of information, but do not do the recovery for the child.

Another teaching technique is to walk around an area (a yard, house, or school), pretending that you are lost and need the child to guide you to "home base." Follow whatever directions the child gives and help the youngster attend to any sensory information that will help in the formulation of a plan. Each time you play, go a little farther from home base.

Travel devices

Cane. Of the travel devices that help a blind traveler safely gather information about the environment, the long cane is the most common. Cane lengths vary as they are "prescribed." As the child grows, the cane length will need to be increased so it informs the child of what is at least two full steps ahead of him. After instruction in the proper use of the cane by an orientation and mobility specialist, the child is able to detect most obstacles in his path and detect such dropoffs as curbs and stairs. The child should be encouraged to travel in areas that the orientation and mobility instructor has stated the child can negotiate safely and independently.

Optical devices. Some visually impaired children with remaining vision can use the telescope for travel. When the telescopic device is prescribed by an optical specialist

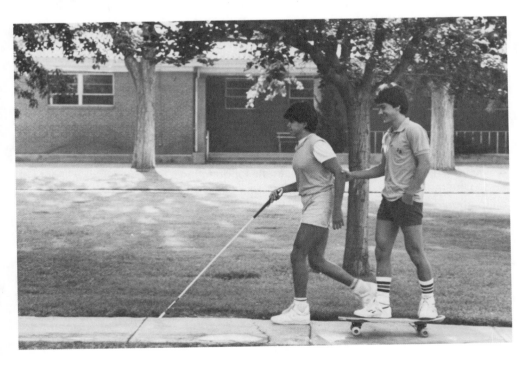

and the child has been instructed in its use by an orientation and mobility specialist, it can be used to locate landmarks, to read street signs, to watch for signal lights, and to read house numbers. Adults can reinforce the use of this device by reminding the child to focus as necessary, to use a support to steady the image, and to scan systematically when searching for an object. Communication among the child's parents, teachers, and the orientation and mobility specialist is essential if the child is to use the telescope properly.

Electronic devices. Electronic devices use auditory or vibration signals to provide information about the nature and location of obstacles and other objects. Because the devices (Sonic Guide, Laser Cane, Mowat Sensor) are in various stages of development and tend to be costly, they should be used only when recommended and taught by an orientation and mobility specialist who is trained in the specific device in question. The devices allow the child to detect clues in the environment but do not replace other orientation and mobility techniques. Some are used in conjunction with a cane or guide dog.

Guide dogs. Blind adolescents and adults may benefit from a guide dog, but they must have good orientation skills because they must direct the dog. Generally, schools that provide guide dog training do not accept students until they are in high school or have graduated from high school because the mastery of orientation and mobility skills is a factor in maintaining a disciplined working relationship with the guide dog.

Maps. If the child is able to use maps, adults can make simple tactile maps using cardboard, sandpaper, or string to show the layout of a classroom or a friend's house. Have the child use the map to determine how to go from point to point. It should be understood that the ability to conceptualize a tactile map is learned gradually and depends on the child's level of development. For example, maps may be very simple at first, showing the child's room or classroom, and progress to her house or apartment, to the block where home is located, to multiple block areas, to small business districts and so forth.

Public places. The lack of vision or inexperience with independent travel should not restrict the child's opportunities to travel in public places. The child needs experience in traveling to and within stores, malls, airports, train and bus stations, restaurants, movie theaters, post offices, and other public areas to increase his awareness and to gain confidence. The child should be actively involved in the purpose of a particular trip, placing an order in a restaurant, purchasing an item while conversing with a sales clerk, making a deposit at a bank, bringing in shoes for repair, asking for a ticket at a ticket counter, or asking fellow pedestrians for directions. Such activities will not only add to the reality of the situation but will expand the child's learning experiences. The child should also participate in routine daily activities in the community.

Transportation systems. Transportation systems should be explored by and explained to young visually impaired children. Let them become familiar with the interior and exterior of automobiles and explain how they operate. Take bus, train, and subway rides, letting the youngster become familiar with the structure of these vehicles and how to pay the fares. Identify each stop with the child. These early experiences provide a background for expanded travel skills.

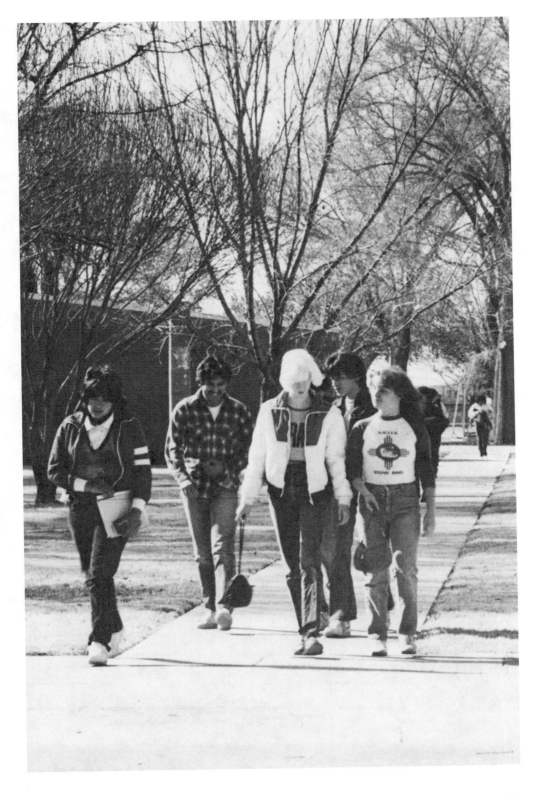

Part III
LEISURE AND RECREATIONAL ACTIVITIES

INTRODUCTION

Blind and visually impaired children need to be guided in the productive use of their leisure time. When they are young, they need to be shown how to play independently and with other children and they must have outdoor experiences—moving, tumbling, and running in open space; feeling sand with their feet and fingers; and stomping in puddles.

Play is the wellspring of imagination. Adults should help visually impaired children discover activities they can enjoy independently. Four-year-old children may not be ready to learn to bowl or skate, but they can learn to run, swim, or to move their bodies in creative movements to music—activities that provide a foundation for the development of later skills. Skiing, dancing, hiking, choral singing, playing a musical instrument, and going on group outings expand the children's horizons, provide opportunities to meet new friends, and help them to be a part of the world around them.

It should be pointed out that personal skills are interrelated with leisure activities. These skills, which have been discussed throughout the previous sections of this manual, include posture and motor development, travel skills, communication skills, dining skills, money management, and the efficient use of vision. It is necessary for a child to develop these skills so that his behavior is socially acceptable. The participation in leisure activities is a practical way of applying these previously learned skills.

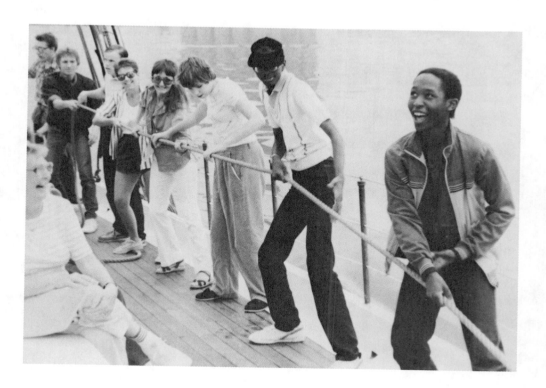

ELEMENTS OF RECREATIONAL EDUCATION

To be able to use their free time appropriately and to build skills for a lifetime of recreational pleasure, blind and visually impaired children and the adults who guide them should experience the four elements of recreational education: 1) awareness of leisure activities, 2) the development of the recreational skills, 3) the determination of an interest inventory, and 4) the exploration and use of resources.

Awareness of leisure activities

Blind and visually impaired children should learn which types of leisure activities, both individual and group, are available to make life enjoyable and sometimes more productive. Their experiences should be so constructed that they have and enjoy the challenge of trying new activities. As they learn to do new things and develop further, they are able to choose among many recreational activities throughout their lives.

Helping sighted individuals become aware of the capabilities of visually impaired children is another aspect of awareness. Although scout leaders, swimming instructors, or community recreation leaders may have heard of blind and visually impaired people who ride horseback, bowl, golf, and so forth, they may never have met such persons. Thus, they need some help in teaching specific recreational skills to children who cannot see well enough to learn through imitation. This help or guidance should be available from specialists such as rehabilitation teachers, special education teachers, parents and, in some instances, the children themselves.

Development of recreational skills

During their school years, blind and visually impaired children can and should be exposed to and participate in a wide variety of indoor and outdoor activities. They need to be directed in these activities so they become familiar with the materials, procedures, rules, and skills required for various activities. These youngsters can learn to participate in table games, such as cards, chess, Scrabble, Parcheesi, Bingo, and checkers; in active sports, such as swimming, bicycling, skiing, softball, and soccer; and as spectators in activities such as professional baseball and football. Eventually, with help and experience, they will choose and engage in self-selected and self-directed activities.

All children need to learn how to win or lose graciously. To do so, they should be given opportunities to experience realistic win/lose situations, both of which are part of playing games. Whenever competition is involved, there are always winners and losers. Children test their skills through competitive games and sports. Blind and visually impaired children should be afforded the same opportunities to engage in competitive activities when they are emotionally ready to do so.

Age-appropriate activities. Many factors are to be considered in determining what is an age-appropriate activity. One factor is the child's chronological, not mental age; thus, an activity is age-appropriate if sighted peers who are the same chronological

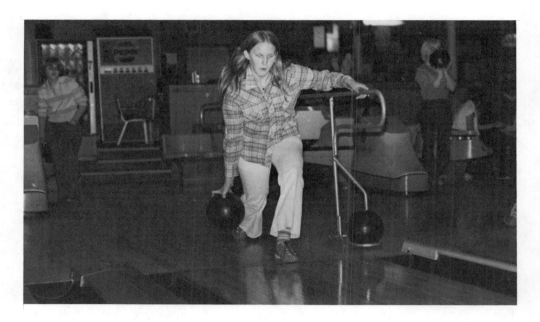

age participate in it in the same or a like situation. Circumstances also determine the appropriateness of an activity. For example, a 5-year-old may make sand castles at the seashore, alongside a group of college students who are doing the same thing, and both could be considered to be performing an age-appropriate activity. But a 16-year-old who is playing alone with a shovel and pail could hardly be considered to be engaging in age-appropriate play.

Other factors involved in the determination of age appropriateness include the child's level of vision, previous experiences, and likes and dislikes. The child should be helped to choose activities according to the degree of difficulty they present. The activities should be challenging but not overwhelming, interesting, and pleasurable. The child should gain satisfaction from her accomplishments. If an activity is competitive, the child should feel gratified, regardless of whether she wins or loses.

Suggested arts and crafts activities

Pudding painting	Paper collages
Finger painting	Soap carving
Mud pies	Self-molding clay
Drawing	Macrame
Clay modeling	Crocheting
Papier-mâché	Knitting
Pasting	Model building
Cutting	String art
Crayon rubbings	Caning
Paper weaving	Loom weaving
Soap drawings	Sculpture

Suggested cultural outings

Circuses
Children's petting zoos
Puppet shows
Firehouses
Train stations
Bakeries
Pet stores

Sensory gardens
Museums
Plays
Concerts
Ice shows
Spectator sports

Suggested social events

Family weddings
School dances

Community picnics

Suggested drama activities

Listening to stories
Imitating sounds and body
  movements of animals

Finger plays and action songs
Writing plays
Performing in plays

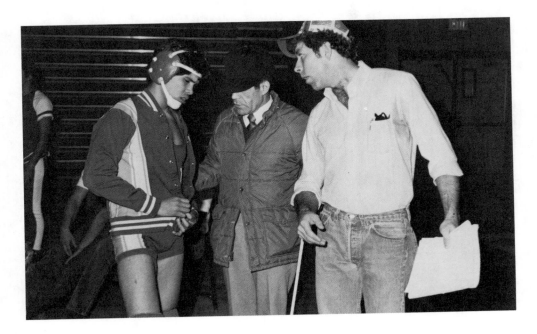

Suggested dance activities
Rhythm games
Marching and clapping
Exercises and movement to music
Popular dancing
Break dancing

Folk and square dancing
Tap, ballet, and modern dance
Performing in dance recitals
Attending school dances and
  proms

Suggested musical activities
Clapping
Listening
Singing
Rhythm band

Instrumental music lessons
Performing in recitals, school
  musicals, orchestras, and
  marching bands

Suggested hobbies
Collecting buttons, rocks, coins,
  and so forth
Playing with dolls
Painting

Cooking
Ham radio
Sewing

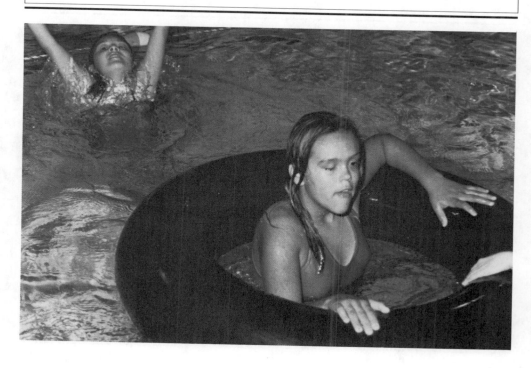

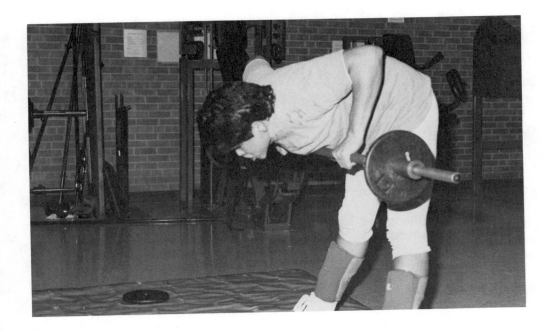

Suggested board games and puzzles

Bingo

Checkers

Chess

Monopoly

Life

Scrabble

Large-type crossword puzzles

Suggested community service

Volunteer work

Performing

Membership in clubs

Debating

Fund raising

Suggested water activities

Bathing

Splashing and kicking

Water play

Swimming and floating

Rowing a boat

Snorkeling

Rafting

Paddling a canoe

Water skiing

Sailing

Rafting

Suggested outdoor/nature study activities

Walking
Climbing
Swinging
Making snow sculptures
Sledding
Bike riding

Gardening
Animal and plant study
Hiking
Horseback riding
Skiing (cross country and
   downhill)

Suggested literary activities

Visits to the library
Reading
Writing letters and
   thank-you notes
Interviewing people

Reporting the news
Writing news stories, analyses,
   and commentaries
Writing short stories, poetry,
   limericks, and jokes

Suggested games

Tag
Hot potato
Drop the hankie
Over-under ball
Duck, duck, goose

Cat and mouse
Dodge ball
Red rover
Fox and geese
Simon says

Suggested playground activities

Sandbox
Swinging
Sliding

Climbing
Riding a merry-go-round
Jumping rope

Suggested sports

Bowling
Kickball
Softball
Basketball
Roller skating

Ice skating
Golf
Tennis
Skiing (cross country and
   downhill)

Adaptations

If a visually impaired or blind child does not receive enough satisfaction from an activity to maintain his interest, it may be that the activity, rules, and materials are not suitable for someone with limited or no vision, and may need to be modified.

Ways to modify activities
Use of sighted partners
Guide ropes
Rails

Sounds
Items of different textures and
distinct color contrast

Many games, such as playing cards, checkers, Scrabble, and Monopoly, come in braille and large-type versions.

The goal of an activity may also be modified to accommodate the child. For example, instead of the game ending when one person attains a certain score, the rules may be changed so the game is over after a specified time has elapsed. Rules may be adjusted to allow for slower or decreased movements, greater repetition, increased time periods, or the incorporation of a buddy system.

The objective of modifying an activity is to allow the child to play as independently as possible without losing the significance of the activity. If too many adjustments are required, it may be necessary to select a different activity. Do not assume that an activity needs to be modified. Rather, begin by instructing the child in the necessary skills. If a particular aspect of the game is overwhelming or cannot be performed without some modification, then adapt the activity to the child's or group's particular needs.

Inventory of interests

Assessment. There are several assessment approaches that may help a child determine her present and anticipated future leisure and recreation needs and abilities and develop a process for carrying out a personal life-long program of leisure activities. After making such an assessment, the child and adult are able to identify the child's interests and to locate accessible leisure programs.

Three ways to determine the recreational needs and abilities of visually impaired children are suggested. The first approach, a checklist, requires that the child, during an interview with his parents and teachers, identify from a list those activities in which he is active and those in which he would like to become involved. During the interview, the interviewer may wish to evaluate the extent or limitations of the child's experiences and the reliability of the responses. The second approach is an interview or discussion session with the child, parents, and teacher in which the child's likes and dislikes of certain types of activities are considered. Suggested activities are then described and discussed. The third approach is to observe the child during individual and group play. By noting a child's play activities, the observer is able to identify the child's apparent interests and abilities. This approach may not be reliable because the children may have had only limited experiences. Thus, the observer may be noting the child's lack of experience, rather than the lack of desire to participate. Ideally, a combination of assessment approaches should be used.

To pinpoint the child's leisure behaviors, concerned adults can use the three approaches to help determine activity areas from which the child gains the most satisfaction and enjoyment—the basis for developing useful skills. As the child grows and gains in experience through exposure to a greater number of activities, adults should encourage the child to explore new activity areas and engage in self-directed activities.

A record of the child's interests should be kept. This file identifies the activities in which the child has participated and those in which she would like to participate, given the opportunity. It identifies what the child can do, as well as what she would like to do during free time. It should also serve as an indicator of those activities to which the child should be exposed because she has no experience with them.

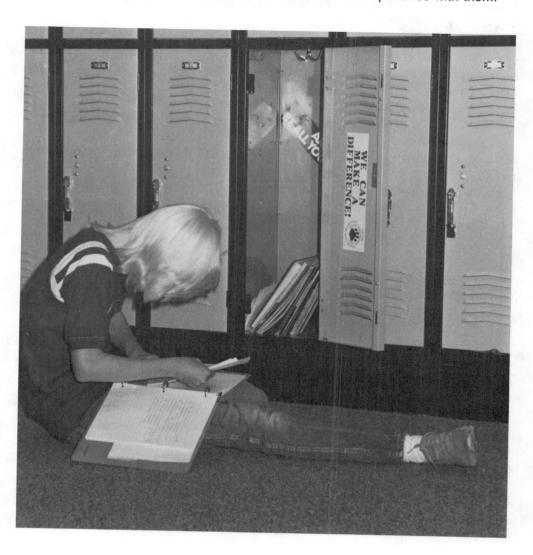

Counseling. Through counseling, adults help the child select activities for the present and plan for the future. The information acquired during assessment is now used to develop a realistic plan of recreational activities. At first, adults assume a direct role in helping the child to become aware of leisure activities. As the child gains leisure skills and is able to make independent decisions, adults become less directive and more supportive or advisory.

Initially, adults are the link from the child's desire and need for activities to the available resources. As the child matures, he must update his own leisure file and explore or further develop interests. The eventual goal of counseling is the child's development of skills and motivation necessary to sustain a leisure activity program throughout life.

Planning the child's leisure time

Listen to records or tapes of children playing.

Read stories to the child.

Walk to parks and play areas, toy stores, and shopping malls.

List activities and question the child about activities in which she would like to take part.

Ask the child, "What would you like to do for fun?"

Observe which activities stimulate the senses.

Show or describe to the child pictures and slides of children playing or participating in outside activities.

Make suggestions to the child.

After the child plays with other children, ask questions:

"What did you play?"

"How did you feel after you did it?"

"Were you glad you did it?"

"Why were you glad you did it?"

Reinforce a child's play by talking with the child after the game or keeping a record of her activities.

Stimulate the child's awareness by asking questions:

"Did you do anything interesting?"

"Why did you like the activity?"

Have the child keep a record of activities during one 24-hour period.

Visit parts of the community or take a walk and record the child's "I want to do's" on index cards.

Have a family or group discussion to help the participants discover each other's interests.

Schedule a specific time each day or week to plan leisure activities for the coming day or week.

Maintain a bulletin board in the family's recreation room that includes a calendar (large type or braille) of coming events, a time clock of daily activities, and a list of the child's "I like to do" statements.

Read magazines, newspapers, advertisements, and books that include things to do around town.

Encourage the child to keep a written or taped diary of her leisure experiences.

Take field trips and visits to sports events, musuem exhibits, and various kinds of performances.

Make a memory book that includes pictures, tickets, dried leaves and flowers, and programs.

Talk with other parents and teachers to learn what other children are doing.

Exploration and use of resources

The leisure activities that are available through the schools and community agencies, as well as at home, may be determined by mailing survey forms to agencies, making a checklist of personal resources, calling community contacts, and meeting with administrators. The end result is a list of local leisure programs. Catalogs or files that describe the content, cost, location, and schedules of programs, adaptations offered for blind and visually impaired children, requirements for participation, and transportation arrangements should also be obtained. Then, the child, with the help of adults, can match her interests with the available resources.

Integration into community programs. Most agencies or organizations do not provide group activities or facilities specifically for blind or visually impaired children. Therefore, the children should be integrated into available recreational programs that are provided for sighted children of the same age.

Two types of preparation will ease a child's successful integration into community programs. First, the adult should visit representative personnel of local agencies or organizations to discuss their attitudes toward the child's participation, the functional level and leisure needs of the child, and the child's previous experiences. Adaptations of activities and equipment should also be discussed, if applicable to the situation. When the child is old enough, he should take on these responsibilities. Second, the child needs to prepare to participate in the new activity. He must apply already-learned skills and learn new ones that are unique to the new activity, anticipate the social skills required by the situation and act accordingly, and deal effectively with new acquaintances who may demonstrate both positive and negative attitudes toward blindness or visual impairment.

Many agencies that provide leisure services offer both individual and group activities. Some agencies provide referral services, such as the Red Cross, which refers individuals to water safety programs suitable to their needs. Community resources include YM-YWCA or YM-YWHAs, local departments of recreation and parks, the Boy and Girl Scouts, religious groups, private agencies, special-interest clubs, children's theater groups, civic groups, and agencies that provide services specifically for disabled persons.

It is important to prepare the child for success. Over the years, the child should have learned how to interact effectively with others, how to utilize socially appropriate behaviors, and how to establish positive social contacts with peers. Usually, success in recreational and leisure activities is due more to social factors than to the child's developmental level. The parents and other adults must continually guide and encourage the child to participate in a variety of experiences and situations that will enrich and expand the child's life. In addition, the child must be able to travel safely and independently from home to wherever the recreational or leisure activity is offered. Having done so, the child has acquired the skills to thrive, not just to survive.

FOR FURTHER READING

Daily living skills

"Academics Are Not Enough: Techniques of Daily Living for Visually Impaired Children," by D.W. Tuttle, 1981, *Handbook for Teachers of the Visually Handicapped*, American Printing House for the Blind, Louisville, KY.

An Analysis of U.S. Sex Education Programs and Evaluation Methods, by D. Kirby, J. Alter & P. Scales, 1979, Report No. CDC-2021-79-DK-FR, U.S. Dept. of Health, Education and Welfare, Washington, DC.

A Resource Guide for Parents and Educators of Blind Children, by D.M. Willoughby, 1979, National Federation of the Blind, Baltimore, MD.

A Step-By-Step Guide to Personal Management for Blind Persons, 1974, American Foundation for the Blind, Inc., New York, NY.

A Study of the Treatment of Blindisms Using Punishment and Positive Reinforcement in Laboratory and Natural Settings, by B. Blasch, 1975, unpublished doctoral dissertation, Michigan State University.

"A Taxonomy for Mannerisms of Blind Children," by V.J. Eichel, 1979, *Journal of Visual Impairment & Blindness*, 73(5) pp. 167-168.

Becoming Me: A Personal Adjustment Guide for Secondary Students, by T. Throckmorton, 1980, Grand Rapids Public Schools, Grand Rapids, MI.

"Behavioral Treatment of Aggression and Self-Injury in Developmentally Disabled, Visually Handicapped Students," by J.K. Luiselli & R.L. Michaud, 1983, *Journal of Visual Impairment & Blindness*, 77(8), pp. 388-392.

Belonging, by D. Kent, 1978, The Dial Press, New York, NY.

Beyond Words, by R.P. Harrison, 1974, Prentice-Hall, Englewood Cliffs, NJ.

Bibliographies of Holdings of the SIECUS Information Service & Library: Sexuality and Illness, Disability, or Aging, by L. Hallingby, 1982, SIECUS, New York, NY.

"Blindisms: Some Observations and Propositions," by L.T. Hoshmand, 1975, *Education of the Visually Handicapped*, 3, pp. 37-40.

Bodily Communication, by M. Argyle, 1975, International Universities Press, New York, NY.

Body Language, by J. Fast, 1970, M. Evans, New York, NY.

"Clothing as Communication," by L.B. Rosenfeld & T.G. Plax, 1977, *Journal of Communication*, 27, pp. 24-31.

"Communication by Facial Expression," by F. Williams & J. Tolch, 1965, *Journal of Communication*, 15, pp. 17-21.

"Daily Living Skills," by P.H. Campbell, 1977, *Developing Individualized Education Programs for Severely Handicapped Children and Youth*, Bureau of Education for the Handicapped, U.S. Dept. of Health, Education & Welfare, Washington, DC.

"Development of Personal Space Schemata," by M. Meisels & C. Guardo, 1969, *Child Development*, 40, pp. 1167-1178.

"Differential Assessments of Blindisms," by M.A. Smith, M. Chetnik & E. Adelson, 1969, *American Journal of Orthopsychiatry*, 39, pp. 807-817.

"Do Blind Children Need Sex Education?," by E. Foulke & T. Unde, 1975, *Sex Education for the Visually Handicapped in Schools and Agencies, Selected Papers*, American Foundation for the Blind, Inc., New York, NY.

"Everyone, Everywhere, Everyday Needs the Tools of the Trade Called Living: Home Economics/Daily Living Skills Assessment, 1985, Nebraska School for the Visually Handicapped, Nebraska City, NE.

"Experimental Attempts to Reduce Stereotyping Among Blind Students," by D. Guess & G. Rutherford, 1967, *Journal of Mental Deficiency*, 71, pp. 984-986.

"Extinguishing Blindisms: A Paradigm of Intervention," by B.S. Miller and W.H. Miller, 1976, *Education of the Visually Handicapped*, 8(1), pp. 6-15.

"Eye Rubbing in Blind Children: Application of a Sensory Deprivation Model," by R. Thurell & D. Rice, 1970, *Exceptional Children*, 36, pp. 325-330.

Feeling Good About Yourself: A Guide for People Working with People Who Have Disabilities, by G. Blum & G. Blum, 1981, Second Edition, Feeling Good Associates, California.

"Finding a Way Through the Rough Years: How Blind Girls Survive Adolescence," by D. Kent, 1983, *Journal of Visual Impairment & Blindness*, 77(7), pp. 247-249.

Housekeeping Skills: Self-Study Course, by A. Yeadon & L. Newman, 1980, Center for Independent Living, New York, NY.

"How to Deal with Blindisms," by L. Holland, 1971, *Long Cane News*, 4(5), pp. 24-27.

Human Sexuality in Health and Illness, by N.F. Woods, 1984, Third Edition, C.V. Mosby, St. Louis, MO.

Living with Impaired Vision: An Introduction, by A. Yeadon & D. Grayson, 1979, American Foundation for the Blind, Inc., New York, NY.

"Mannerisms in the Congenitally Blind Child," by J. Knight, 1972, *New Outlook for the Blind*, 66 (9), pp. 297-302.

"Mannerisms, Not Blindisms," by J. Morse, 1965, *International Journal for the Education of the Blind*, 15(1), pp. 12-16.

"Mannerisms of the Blind: A Review of the Literature," by V.J. Eichel, 1978, *Journal of Visual Impairment & Blindness*, 72, pp. 125-130.

"Modification of Manneristic Behavior in a Visually Impaired Child Via a Time-Out Procedure," by R.L. Simpson, G.M. Sasso & N. Bump, 1982, *Education of the Visually Handicapped*, 14(2), pp. 50-55.

Non-Verbal Communication Through Touch, by A.I. Smith, 1970, unpublished doctoral dissertation, Georgia State University.

Openness to Touching: A Study of Strangers in Nonverbal Interaction, by D.N. Walker, 1971, unpublished doctoral dissertation, University of Connecticut.

"Procedures Used to Modify Self-Injurious Behaviors in Visually Impaired, Mentally Retarded Individuals," by J. Longo, A.F. Rotatori, G. Kapperman & T. Heinze, 1981, *Education of the Visually Handicapped*, 13(3) pp. 77-83.

"Programs in Daily Living Skills," by E. Schultz, 1968, *Association for Education of the Visually Handicapped Forty-Ninth Biennial Conference Proceedings*, Toronto, Ontario, Canada.

"Reduction of Rocking Mannerisms in Two Blind Children," by A. Caetano & J. Kauffman, 1975, *Education of the Visually Handicapped*, 7(4), pp. 101-105.

"Retrolental Fibroplasia and Autistic Symptomology," by J.B. Chase, 1972, *Research Series No. 24*, American Foundation for the Blind, Inc., New York, NY.

Sewing, by J. Crane, 1978, Center for Independent Living, New York, NY.

Sex and Disability: A Resource Guide to Books, Pamphlets, Articles, and Audio, Visual and Tactile Materials, by E. Smith, P. Silver & K. Hughes, 1981, Planned Parenthood, Alameda/San Francisco, CA.

Sex Education and Family Life for Visually Handicapped Children and Youth: A Resource Guide, by I.R. Dickman, 1975, SIECUS and American Foundation for the Blind, Inc., New York, NY.

"Sex Education of Blind Children," by F. van'T Hooft & K. Heslinga, 1975, *Sex Education for the Visually Handicapped in Schools and Agencies . . . Selected Papers*, American Foundation for the Blind, Inc., New York, NY.

"Sexuality and the Family Life Span," 1982, *Proceedings from Changing Family Conference XI*, University of Iowa, Division of Continuing Education, Iowa City, IA.

"Sexuality During Adolescence," by P.H. Dreyer, 1982, *Handbook of Developmental Psychology*, edited by B.B. Wolman & G. Stricker, Prentice Hall, Englewood Cliffs, NJ.

"Social Skills," by K.M. Huebner, 1986, *Foundations of Education for Blind and Visually Handicapped Children and Youth: Theory and Practice*, edited by G.T. Scholl, American Foundation for the Blind, Inc., New York, NY.

"Social Skills Training of a Blind Child Through Differential Reinforcement," by G.M. Farkas, R.B. Sherick, J.C. Matson & M. Loebig, 1981, *The Behavior Therapist*, 4, pp. 24-26.

Teacher Workbook for Family Life Education, S.E. Knight & C.E. Thornton, 1983, Document No. ED 229-685, ERIC Documents Reproduction Service.

Techniques of Daily Living: A Curriculum Guide, by M.E. Wehrum, 1977, The Greater Pittsburgh Guild for the Blind, Bridgeville, PA.

"The Availability of Sex Education in Large City Schools," by F.L. Sonenstein & K.J. Pittman, 1984, *Family Planning Perspectives* 16(1), pp. 19-25.

"The Effects of Furniture Arrangement, Props, and Personality on Social Interaction," by A. Mehrabian & S.G. Diamond, 1971, *Journal of Personality and Social Psychology*, 20, pp. 18-30.

The Emerging Male: A Man's Handbook, by R. Crutcher, M. Chaton & L. Koser, 1982, Everyman's Center, California.

"The Expressive Behavior of the Blind-and-Deaf-Born," by I. Eibl-Eibesfeldt, 1975, *Social Communication and Movement*, edited by M. Cranach & I. Vine, Academic Press, New York, NY.

"The Influence of Visual and Ambulation Restrictions on Stereotyped Behavior," by D. Guess, 1966, *Journal of Mental Deficiency*, 70, pp. 542-547.

The Pleasure of Eating for Those Who Are Visually Impaired, by S. Mangold, 1978, Exceptional Teaching Aids, Castro Valley, CA.

"The Psychosocial Effects of Blindness: Implications for Program Planning in Sex Education," by G.T. Scholl, 1975, *Sex Education for the Visually Handicapped in Schools and Agencies . . . Selected Papers*, American Foundation for the Blind, Inc., New York, NY.

"The Significance of Posture in Communicative Systems," by A.E. Scheflen, 1964, *Psychiatry*, 27, pp. 316-331.

"Training Blind Adolescents in Social Skills," by V.R. Van Hasselt, M. Hersen, A.E. Kasdin, J. Simon & A.K. Mastantuono, 1983, *Journal of Visual Impairment & Blindness*, 77(5), pp. 199-203.

Training in Daily Living Skills and Its Effects on the Self Concept of Visually Impaired Children, by S.M. McMakin, 1976, unpublished doctoral dissertation, University of South Carolina.

Verbalism Among Blind Children, by R.K. Harley, 1963, *Research Series No. 10*, American Foundation for the Blind, Inc., New York, NY.

"Visual Behavior and Face-To-Face Distance During Interaction," by G.N. Goldberg, C.A. Kiesler & B.A. Collins, 1969, *Sociometry,* 32, pp. 43-53.

"Visual Defect Does Not Produce Stereotyped Movement" by G. Berkson, 1973, *American Journal of Mental Deficiency*, 78, pp. 89-94.

Who Cares? A Handbook on Sex Education and Counseling Services for Disabled People by S. Chipouras, D. Cornelius, S. Daniels & E. Makas, 1982, Second Edition University Park Press, Baltimore, MD.

Large print and braille materials

Large Print Birth Control Information Sheets (n.d.), Planned Parenthood, Alameda/San Francisco, CA.

Growing Up and Liking It, 1980, Personal Products Co., Milltown, NJ.

For Boys: A Book About Girls, 1980, Personal Products Co., Milltown, NJ.

Birth Control: All the Methods That Work and the Ones That Don't (n.d.), Planned Parenthood, New York, NY. Braille edition,1977, Iowa Commission for the Blind, Des Moines, IA. Large printed edition, 1977, Foundation for Blind Children, Scottsdale, AZ.

Constructed models

Gender Dolls/Models of Human Genital Anatomy
Jim Jackson and Co.
33 Richdale Avenue
Cambridge, MA 02140

Orientation and mobility

"A Concept Development Program for Future Mobility Training," by R. Webster,1976, *New Outlook for the Blind,* 70(5) pp. 195-197.

"Developmental Concepts of Blind Children Between the Ages of Three and Six as They Relate to Orientation and Mobility," by L. Hapeman, 1976, *The International Journal for the Education of the Blind,* 17(2), pp. 41-48.

"Dog Guides," by R.H. Whitstock, 1980, *Foundations of Orientation and Mobility,* edited by R.L. Welsh & B.B. Blasch, American Foundation for the Blind, Inc., New York, NY.

Foundations of Orientation and Mobility, edited by R.L. Welsh & B.B. Blasch, 1980, American Foundation for the Blind, Inc., New York, NY.

"Mobility Devices," by L.W. Farmer, 1980, *Foundations of Orientation and Mobility,* edited by R.L. Welsh and B.B. Blasch, American Foundation for the Blind, Inc., New York, NY.

"Mobility Differences Between Blind Children in Day School and Residential School Settings," by A.E. Blackhurst & C.H. Marks, 1977, *Education of the Visually Handicapped,* 9(3), pp. 85-91.

"Orientation Aids," by B.L. Bentzen, 1980, *Foundations of Orientation and Mobility,* edited by R.L. Welsh & B.B. Blasch, American Foundation for the Blind, Inc., New York, NY.

"Orientation and Mobility for Preschool Children: What We Have and What We Need," by K.A. Ferrell, 1980, *Journal of Visual Impairment & Blindness,* 72(2). pp. 59-66.

Orientation and Mobility Techniques: A Guide for the Practitioner by E.W. Hill & P. Ponder, 1976, American Foundation for the Blind, Inc., New York, NY.

"Relationship Between Mobility Level and Development of Positional Concepts in Visually Impaired Children," by S.E. Miller, 1982, *Journal of Visual Impairment & Blindness,* 76(5), pp. 149-153.

"The Formation of Concepts Involved in Body Position in Space," by E.W. Hill, 1970, *Education of the Visually Handicapped,* 2(4), pp. 112-114.

"The Formation of Concepts Involved in Body Position in Space," Part II, by E.W. Hill, 1971, *Education of the Visually Handicapped,* 3(1), pp. 21-24.

Leisure and recreational activities

"Adapted Canoeing for the Handicapped," by G.H. Frith & L.D. Warren, 1984, *Teaching Exceptional Children,* pp. 219-221.

Adapted Physical Education and Recreation: A Multidisciplinary Approach, by C. Sherrill, 1976, Wm. C. Brown, Dubuque, IA.

"A New Adventure for the Blind: Sailing Without Sight," by R. Hale, 1976, *The Lion,* 59(5), pp.16-17.

Aquatic Recreation for the Blind, by H.C. Cordellos, 1976, Physical Education and Recreation for the Handicapped Information and Research Utilization Center.

"Art for the Blind and Partially Seeing," by C.R. Jones, 1961, *Seeing Arts*, 60, pp. 21-22.

"Athletics for Visually Handicapped Participants," by D. Craft, 1981, *Nautilus Magazine* 3(5), pp. 22-23.

"A Walking-Jogging Program for Blind Persons," by S. Laughlin, 1975, *New Outlook for the Blind*, 69(1), pp. 312-313.

"Ball Games for Visually Handicapped Children," by R.E. Hartman, 1974, *New Outlook for the Blind*, 68(8), pp. 348-355.

"Bicycle Riding Practices of Blind and Partially Sighted Children," by J.D. McNaughton, 1971, *The Chronicle*, 11(7), pp. 6-7.

"Blind Horsemanship," by E.M. Amphlett, 1969, *New Beacon*, 53(621), pp. 4-6.

"Blind Skiing: Cross Country," by O. Miller, 1976, *Journal of Physical Education & Recreation*, 47, pp. 63-64.

"Blind Students Learn Karate," by D. Fisher, 1972, *Journal of Rehabilitation* 38(4), pp. 26-27.

"Blindness and Yoga," by A.D. Heyes, 1974, *New Outlook for the Blind*, 68(9), pp. 385-393.

"Cross Country Running for Visually Impaired Adults," by J.J. Sonka & M.J. Bina, 1978, *Journal of Visual Impairment & Blindness*, 72(6), pp. 212-214.

Dance and the Blind Child, by A. Chapman & M. Cramer, 1973, American Dance Guild, Inc., New York, NY.

"Fencing as an Aid to the Habilitation or Rehabilitation of Blind Persons," by J. Waffa, 1963, *New Outlook for the Blind*, 57(2), pp. 39-43.

"Goal Ball," by S. Kearney & R. Copland, 1979, *Journal of Physical Education*, 2, pp. 24-26.

"Guidelines for Teaching Arts and Crafts to Blind Children in the Elementary Grades," by V.H. Coombs, 1967, *International Journal for the Education of the Blind*, 16, pp. 79-83.

Instructional Manual for Blind Bowlers, by J.E. Zok, 1970, American University and American Blind Bowling Assn., Washington, DC.

Physical Education and Recreation for the Visually Handicapped by C.E. Buell, 1982, revised edition, The American Alliance for Health, Physical Education, Recreation and Dance, Reston, VA.

"Recreation Programming for Visually Impaired Children," by M. Carter & J.D. Kelley, 1981, *Recreation Programming for Visually Impaired Children and Youth*, edited by J.D. Kelley, American Foundation for the Blind, Inc., New York, NY.

Recreation Programming for Visually Impaired Children and Youth, by J.D. Kelley & I. Ludwig, 1984, American Foundation for the Blind, Inc., New York, NY.

"Sailing: A New Experience," by R. DiMattia, 1970, *New Outlook for the Blind*, 64(5), pp. 138-141.

"Sailing Without Sight," by C. Christensen, 1975, *Dialogue*, 14(2), pp. 77-78.

"Skating for the Sightless," by J. Bellinger, 1971, *Rehabilitation Teacher*, 3(3), pp. 23-25.

Strategies for Developing Individualized Recreation/Leisure Plans for Adolescent and Young Adult Severely Handicapped Students, by A. Ford, L. Brown, I. Pumpian, D. Baumgart, J. Schroeder & R. Loomis, 1981, Madison Metropolitan School District, Madison, WI.

"Teaching Blind Beginners How to Ski," by G. Deschamps, 1969, *Rehabilitation Bulletin*, 19, pp. 8-10.

"Teaching the Blind Student Archery Skills," by D. Hyman, 1969, *Journal of Health, Physical Education, Recreation*, 40, pp. 85-86.

"The Effects of Creative Dance Movement on Large Muscle Control and Balance in Congenitally Blind Children," by A. Duehl, 1973, *Journal of Visual Impairment & Blindness*, 73(4), pp. 127-133.

Miscellaneous

Alive . . . Aware . . . A Person, by R. O'Brien, 1976, Montgomery County Public Schools, Rockville, MD.

A Curriculum Guide for the Development of Body and Sensory Awareness for the Visually Impaired, 1974, Illinois Office of Education, Springfield, IL.

A Difference in the Family, by H. Fetherstone, 1981, Penguin Books, New York, NY.

"An Interview Strategy for Language-Deficient Children," by D. Bricker, D. Ruder & L. Vincent, 1976, *Teaching Special Children*, edited by N. Haring & R. Schuefelbusch, McGraw-Hill, New York, NY.

A Primer of Infant Development, by T.G. Bower, 1977, W.H. Freeman, San Francisco, CA.

A Resource Guide for Parents and Educators of Blind Children by D. Willoughby, 1979, National Federation of the Blind, Baltimore, MD.

"Assessment of Blind Students' Conceptual Understanding," by K.T. Wardell, 1976, *New Outlook for the Blind*, 76(10), pp. 445-446.

"Assumptions About Parental Participation: A Legislative History," by H.R. Turnbull, A.P. Turnbull & A. Wheat, 1982, *Exceptional Education Quarterly*, 3, pp. 1-8.

Beginnings: A Practical Guide for Parents and Teachers of Visually Impaired Babies, by S. Moore, 1985, American Printing House for the Blind, Inc., Louisville, KY.

Being Blind, by R. Marcus, 1981, Hastings House, New York, NY.

"Blind Babies See with Their Ears," by T.G. Bower, 1977, *New Scientist*, 73, pp. 255-257.

Blind Children Learn to Read, by B. Lowenfeld, G.L. Abel & P.H. Hatlen, 1969, Charles C Thomas, Springfield, IL.

Blindness and Early Childhood Development, by D. Warren, 1984, American Foundation for the Blind, Inc., New York, NY.

Can't Your Child See?, by E. Scott, J. Jan, & R. Freeman, second edition, 1985, Pro-Ed Press, Austin, TX.

Career Education for Handicapped Children and Youth, by D.E. Brolin & C.J. Kokaska, 1979, Charles E. Merrill, Columbus, OH.

Christopher—A Silent Life, by M. Brock, 1975, Macmillan-London Ltd. London, England.

Code of Braille Textbook Format Techniques, 1977, American Printing House for the Blind, Louisville, KY.

"Creating With Material Can Be of Value for Young Blind Children," by I.W. Kurzhals, 1961, *International Journal for the Education of the Blind*, 10(3), pp. 75-79.

"Developmental Needs in Blind Infants," by R.F. DuBose, 1976, *New Outlook for the Blind*, 70(2), pp. 49-52.

"Development of Efficiency in Visual Functioning: A Literature Analysis," by N.C. Barraga, M. Collins & J.E. Morris, 1977, *Journal of Visual Impairment & Blindness*, 71(9), pp. 387-391.

"Early Childhood Services for Visually Impaired Children: A Model Program," by R. O'Brien, 1975, *New Outlook for the Blind*, 69(5), pp. 201-206.

"Family Communication Styles and Language Development," by L.S. Kekelis & E.S. Anderson, 1984, *Journal of Visual Impairment & Blindness*, 78(2), pp. 54-65.

Focus on Individualized Programming for the Visually Handicapped: Part II, 1977, Pennsylvania Materials Center for the Visually Handicapped.

Foundations of Education for Blind and Visually Handicapped Children and Youth; Theory and Practice, edited by G. Scholl, 1986, American Foundation for the Blind, Inc., New York, NY.

"Functional Vision Criterion-Referenced Checklists," by L.J. Roessing, 1982, *A Teacher's Guide to Educational Needs of Blind and Visually Handicapped Children*, by S.S. Mangold, American Foundation for the Blind, Inc., New York, NY.

Get a Wiggle On: A Guide for Helping Visually Impaired Children Grow, by S. Raynor & R. Drouillard, 1975, AAHPER Publications, Washington, DC.

Getting Help for a Disabled Child: Advice from Parents, by I.R. Dickman & S. Gordon, 1983, Public Affairs Pamphlet No. 615, Public Affairs Committee, Inc., New York, NY.

"Gross and Fine Motor Development," by L. Chandler, 1979, *The Developmental Resource*, edited by M.A. Cohen & P.J. Gorss, Grune & Stratton, New York, NY.

Guidelines and Games for Teaching Efficient Braille Reading, by M.R. Olson & S. Mangold, 1981, American Foundation for the Blind, Inc., New York, NY.

Handbook for Parents of Preschool Blind Children by I. Davidson, et al., 1976, Ontario Institute for Studies in Education, Toronto, Ontario, Canada.

Heart to Heart, by S. Recchia, 1985, The Blind Children's Center, Los Angeles, CA.

Helping Children Learn to Read, by P.J. Finn, 1985, Random House, New York, NY.

Increased Visual Behavior in Low Vision Children, by N.C. Barraga, 1964, American Foundation for the Blind, Inc., New York, NY.

Language Acquisition in the Blind Child: Normal and Deficient, by A.E. Mills, 1983, College Hill Press, San Diego, CA.

Language Development and Language Disorders, by L. Bloom & M. Lahey, 1978, John Wiley, New York, NY.

"Language Development in Blind Multihandicapped Children: A Model of Co-Active Intervention," by S. Rogow, 1980, *Child Care, Health, and Development*, 6, pp. 301-308.

"Learning by Blind Students Through Active and Passive Listening," by C. Nolan & J. Morris, 1969, *Exceptional Children*, 36(3), pp. 173-186.

"Learning Through Listening: A New Approach," by E.S. Cobb, 1977, *Journal of Visual Impairment & Blindness* 71(5), pp. 206-253.

Listening for the Visually Impaired: A Teaching Manual, by C. Stocker, 1973, Charles C Thomas, Springfield, IL.

Look At Me: A Resource Manual for the Development of Residual Vision in Multiply Impaired Children, by A.J. Smith & K.S. Cote, 1982, Pennsylvania College of Optometry, Philadelphia, PA.

Manual for a Work-Experience Program, by J. Tremble & F. Wilson, 1970, Oak Hill School, Hartford, CT.

"Maximizing Parental Involvement in Programs for Exceptional Children: Strategies for Education and Related Service Personnel," by S. Stile, J. Cole & A. Garner, 1979, *Journal of the Division for Early Childhood*, 1, pp. 68-82.

"Motor Development in Blind Children," by V. Hart, 1983, *Help Me Be Everything I Can Be*, edited by M. Wurster & M.E. Mulholland, American Foundation for the Blind, Inc., New York, NY.

"Motor Development in Congenitally Blind Children," by H.C. Griffin, 1981, *Education of the Visually Handicapped* 7(4), pp. 107-111.

Move It!, by S. Raynor & R. Drouillard, 1977, AAHPER Publications, Washington, DC.

"Parental Professional Interactions," by A. Turnbill, 1983, *Systematic Instruction of the Moderately and Severely Handicapped*, edited by M. Snell, Charles E. Merrill Publishing Co., Columbus, OH.

Parenting Preschoolers: Suggestions for Raising Young Blind and Visually Impaired Children, by K.A. Ferrell, 1984, American Foundation for the Blind, Inc., New York, NY.

Preschool Learning Activities for the Visually Impaired Child: A Guide for Parents, by Illinois Office of the Superintendent of Public Instruction, 1975, National Association for Parents of the Visually Impaired, Inc., Austin, TX.

Raising the Young Blind Child, by S. Karstein, I. Spaulding & B. Scharf, 1980, Human Sciences Press Inc., New York, NY.

Reach Out and Teach, by K.A. Ferrell, 1985, American Foundation for the Blind, Inc., New York, NY.

"Relationships of Parents to Professionals: A Challenge to Professionals," by J. Stotland, 1984, *Journal of Visual Impairment & Blindness*, 78(2), pp. 69-74.

Self-Esteem and Adjusting with Blindness, by D.W. Tuttle, 1984, Charles C Thomas, Springfield, IL.

Sensory Training: A Curriculum Guide, by J. Kimbrough, K. Huebner & L. Lowry, 1976, The Greater Pittsburgh Guild for the Blind, Bridgeville, PA.

Show Me How: A Manual for Parents of Preschool Visually Impaired Children, by M. Brennan, 1982, American Foundation for the Blind, Inc., New York, NY.

"Simon Says," Is Not the Only Game, by B. Leary & M. von Schneden, 1982, American Foundation for the Blind, Inc., New York, NY.

Source Book on Low Vision, by N.C. Barraga & J.E. Morris, 1980, American Printing House for the Blind, Louisville, KY.

"Tactual Development and Its Implications for the Education of Blind Children," by H.C. Griffin & P.J. Gerber, 1982, *Education of the Visually Handicapped*, 13, pp. 116-123.

Talk to Me and *Talk to Me II* by L. Kekelis, 1984, 1985, The Blind Children's Center, Los Angeles, CA.

"Task Analysis of a Complex Assembly Task by the Retarded Blind," by M.W. Gold, 1976, *Exceptional Children*, 43(2), pp. 78-84.

Teacher's Guide for Development of Visual Learning Abilities and Utilization of Low Vision, by N.C. Barraga, 1970, American Printing House for the Blind, Louisville, KY.

Teaching Individuals with Physical and Multiple Disabilities by J.L. Bigge, 1982, Charles E. Merrill, Columbus, OH.

"The Blind Child," by R. Ancona, 1971, *Art for the Exceptional,* edited by C. Alkema, Pruett Publishing Co., Boulder, CO.

"The Blind Child as an Integral Part of the Family and Community," by B. Lowenfeld, 1981, *Berthold Lowenfeld on Blindness and Blind People*, American Foundation for the Blind, Inc., New York, NY.

"The Continuum of Services for Visually Handicapped Students," by N. Bryant, 1984, *Quality Services for Blind and Visually Handicapped Learners*, edited by G. Scholl, Council for Exceptional Children, Reston, VA.

"The Development of Language in the Deaf-Blind Multihandicapped Child: Progression of Instructional Methods," by E. Hammer, 1982, *The Multihandicapped Hearing Impaired*, edited by D. Tweedie & E.H. Scroyer, Gallaudet College Press, Washington, DC.

The Educator's Role in the Prevention and Treatment of Child Abuse and Neglect, by D.D. Broadhurst, 1979, National Center for Child Abuse and Neglect, U.S. Dept. of Health, Education, & Welfare, Washington, DC.

"The Effectiveness of Structured Sensory Training Experiences Prior to Formal Orientation and Mobility Instruction," by R. Mills & D. Adamschick, 1969, *Education of the Visually Handicapped*, 1 (1), pp. 14-21.

"The Influence of Preference of Texture on the Accuracy of Tactile Discrimination," by K.A. Hanninen, 1976, *Education of the Visually Handicapped*, 8 (2), pp. 44-52.

The Road to Freedom: A Guide to Prepare the Blind Child to Travel Independently, by R. Webster, 1977, Katan Publications, Jacksonville, IL.

The Visually Handicapped Child in Your Classroom, by E. Scott, 1977, University Park Press, Baltimore, MD.

Touch the Baby: Blind and Visually Impaired Children as Patients—Helping Them Respond to Care, by L. Harrell, 1984, American Foundation for the Blind, Inc., New York, NY.

Visual Handicaps and Learning, by N. Barraga, 1983, Exceptional Resources, Austin, TX.

Visual Impairment in Children and Adolescents, by J. Jan, R. Freeman, & E. Scott, 1977, Grune & Stratton, New York, NY.

Welcome to the World, by S. Recchia, 1985, The Blind Children's Center, Los Angeles, CA.

Your Child's Sensory World, by L. Liepmann, 1973, Dial Press, New York, NY.

SERVICES AND ORGANIZATIONS

American Council of the Blind
Council of Families with Visual Impairment
1155 15th Street, N.W., Suite 720
Washington, DC 20005
(202) 467-5081 or (800) 424-8666

American Foundation for the Blind
11 Penn Plaza, Suite 300
New York, NY 10001
(212) 502-7600 or (800) 232-5463

American Printing House for the Blind
1839 Franfort Avenue
Louisville, KY 40206
(502) 895-2405 or (800) 223-1839

Association for Education and Rehabilitation
of the Blind and Visually Impaired
4600 Duke Street, Suite 430
Alexandria, VA 22304
(703) 823-8690

The Association for Persons with Severe
Handicaps
29 West Susquehanna Avenue, Suite 210
Baltimore, MD 21204
(410) 828-8274

Blind Children's Fund
2875 North Wind Drive, No. 211
East Lansing, MI 48823
(517) 333-1725

Children's Braille Book-of-the-Month Club
National Braille Press
88 St. Stephen Street
Boston, MA 02115
(617) 266-6160

Council for Exceptional Children
1110 North Glebe Road, Suite 300
Arlington, VA, 22201-5704
(703) 620-3660 or (888) CEC-SPED

Exceptional Teaching Aids
20102 Woodbine Avenue
Castro Valley, CA 94546
(510) 582-4859 or (800) 549-6999

The Foundation Fighting Blindness
Executive Plaza 1, Suite 800
11350 McComick Road
Hunt Valley, MD 21031-1014
(410) 785-1414 or (888) 394-3937

Hadley School for the Blind
700 Elm Street
Winnetka, IL 60093
(847) 446-8111 or (800) 232-4238

Howe Press
Perkins School for the Blind
175 North Beacon Street
Watertown, MA 02172
(617) 924-3490

The John Tracy Clinic
806 West Adams Boulevard
Los Angeles, CA 90007
(213) 748-5481

National Association for Parents of Children
with Visual Impairments
P. O. Box 317
Watertown, MA 02272-0317
(800) 562-6265

National Association for Visually
Handicapped
22 West 21st Street
New York, NY 10010
(212) 889-3141

National Center for Education in Maternal
and Child Health
2000 15th Street North, Suite 701
Arlington, VA 22201-2617
(703) 524-7802

National Library Service for the Blind
and Physically Handicapped
Library of Congress
1291 Taylor Street, N.W.
Washington, DC 20542
(202) 707-5100 or (800) 424-8567

National Organization for Albinism and
Hypopigmentation (NOAH)
1530 Locust Street, No. 29
Philadelphia, PA 19102-4415
(215) 545-2322 or (800) 473-2310

National Organization of Parents of Blind
Children
Division of National Federation of the Blind
1800 Johnson Street
Baltimore, MD 21230
(410) 659-9314

ABOUT THE EDITORS

Rose-Marie Swallow, Ed.D.

now retired, was, at the time of writing, professor and coordinator of the teacher education program for the visually impaired at California State University, Los Angeles. A former teacher of visually handicapped students, she is co-author of *Informal Assessment of Developmental Skills for Visually Handicapped Students* and a contributing author of *Foundations of Education for Blind and Visually Handicapped Children and Youth: Theory and Practice,* as well as author of several articles related to assessment and teaching strategies, instructional programming, and preschool education.

Kathleen Mary Huebner, Ph.D.

is chair of the Department of Graduate Studies in Vision Impairment and director of Education and Rehabilitation Programs at the Institute for the Visually Impaired, Pennsylvania College of Optometry, in Philadelphia. At the time of writing, she was director of national services in education, low vision, and orientation and mobility for the American Foundation for the Blind. She has taught blind and visually impaired children, youths, and adults in a variety of settings and directed the master's degree teacher preparation program at the State University of New York, College of Arts and Science at Geneseo. She is a co-editor of *Hand in Hand: Essentials of Communication and Orientation and Mobility for Your Students Who Are Deaf-Blind* and a contributing author of *Foundations of Education for Blind and Visually Handicapped Children and Youth: Theory and Practice.*